MOSBY'S
TOUR GUIDE TO
NURSING SCHOOL
A Student's Road Survival Kit

In collaboration with NSNA
National Student Nurses' Association, Inc.

MOSBY'S
TOUR GUIDE TO
NURSING SCHOOL
A Student's Road Survival Kit

Melodie Chenevert, *RN, BSN, MN, MA*
Pro-Nurse
Gaithersburg, Maryland

SIXTH EDITION

MOSBY

ELSEVIER

3251 Riverport Lane
Maryland Heights, MO 63043

MOSBY'S TOUR GUIDE TO NURSING SCHOOL:
A STUDENT'S ROAD SURVIVAL KIT   ISBN: 978-0-323-06741-6
Copyright © 2011 by Mosby, Inc., an affiliate of Elsevier Inc.

Notice

Neither the Publisher nor the Author assumes any responsibility for any loss or injury and/or damage to persons or property arising out of or related to any use of the material contained in this book. It is the responsibility of the treating practitioner, relying on independent expertise and knowledge of the patient, to determine the best treatment and method of application for the patient.

The Publisher

Previous editions copyrighted 1987, 1991, 1995, 2002, 2006

Library of Congress Cataloging-in-Publication Data
Chenevert, Melodie, 1941–
    Mosby's tour guide to nursing school : a student's road survival kit / Melodie
Chenevert. — 6th ed.
        p. ; cm.
    Includes bibliographical references and index.
    ISBN 978-0-323-06741-6 (pbk. : alk. paper) 1. Nursing students. 2. Nursing schools. 3. Nursing—Vocational guidance. 4. Success. I. National Student Nurses' Association (U. S.) II. Title. III. Title: Tour guide to nursing school.
    [DNLM: 1. Schools, Nursing—Popular Works. 2. Education, Nursing—Popular Works. 3. Vocational Guidance—Popular Works. WY 19 C518m 2011]
    RT73.C49 2011
    610.73071' 1—dc22   2009043311

Acquisitions Editor: Yvonne Alexopolous
Developmental Editor: Heather Rippetoe
Publishing Services Manager: Jeff Patterson
Project Manager: Jeanne Genz
Design Direction: Amy Buxton

Printed in The United States of America

Last digit is the print number: 9 8 7 6 5

Working together to grow
libraries in developing countries

www.elsevier.com | www.bookaid.org | www.sabre.org

ELSEVIER   BOOK AID International   Sabre Foundation

Dedicated to the future nurse
and
the future of nursing . . .
they are one and the same

Note to Students

When I was invited to write this introduction for the latest edition of Melodie Chenevert's *Mosby's Tour Guide to Nursing School,* I could not have been more excited. I can say with complete honesty that this book has been my go-to text for my last 2 years of nursing school—I only wish that I had found it sooner! When I began nursing school just over 4 years ago, my vision of the journey ahead was foggy at best. I knew so little about nursing as a profession; let alone what to expect in my education. I knew nothing of the tests to come of my memory, intelligence, emotional strength, and integrity. As long as the journey has been, it is the turns I have taken along the highway that have come together to make me who I am today, as I'm sure will be the case for you.

I began nursing school thinking that nursing involved sitting at a patient's bedside all day, providing compassionate care. I knew nothing about having high patient loads, difficult patients, complicated medical cases, loss of a patient, or loss of trust in myself. I didn't anticipate the joy of a patient saying thank you, or a baby being born. It has been a long road through school, but I have come out the other side a stronger and more confident person. I remember being *terrified* during my first clinical. I wondered what would happen if I didn't get the blood pressure right or missed something in a head-to-toe assessment. I stressed over long-term career goals and what specialties I wanted to go into. Today, a head-to-toe assessment is an automatic process, and I've managed to narrow down my long-term professional goals.

I am now in my last semester of BSN education, and have worked part time for the last year at a local hospital's family birthing center in the postpartum department. I love going to work every day, and I'm confident in the patient care that I provide. One of the most common things I hear from my patients in the postpartum unit is, "Why can't children come with a manual?" I'm still working on finding a manual for them, but I can say with confidence that this book is the perfect manual for you and your next several years in school.

Through my work with the National Student Nurses' Association I have seen many students at the beginning of their educational journey. I suggest that they find a mentor who has been through the same journey. This book is your personal mentor in your backpack. Reference it often to learn about next steps, financing, professional aspects of nursing, and much more. I'm not sure I could have made it over the potholes and around the traffic jams of my nursing education without this book! I wish you the very best of luck on your journey. With this book in hand and a love for nursing in your heart, the ride will be over before you know it. Bon voyage!

Jenna Sanders
2008-09 President
National Student Nurses' Association
www.nsna.org

Preface

Now that you have a copy of this book, keep it close at hand.

Before every test, every term paper, every presentation you have to give, re-read the appropriate chapter. It will only take a few moments and the down-to-earth tips can make an average student good and a good student great.

A nursing faculty member shared this example.

"One of my first-semester students failed the first exam in the first clinical course. She was devastated to say the least. I worked with her on study skills and test-taking skills on several occasions. She joined a study group, did flash cards, and even composed questions about the content so she could test herself. One of the things I told her to do was to read the chapters in this book on studying and taking tests as well as the chapter on failure. She read them over and over each day. When the next exam rolled around, she got a B! She was surprised, thrilled, and overjoyed. This particular student continued to read the chapters in this book before each exam. She passed every course and the NCLEX® with flying colors! She is now headed to graduate school."

At a city-wide extravaganza honoring graduating nursing students, a young man glanced at my name tag. "You!" he exclaimed. "You're the person who wrote that book! You're the person who got me through nursing school!" He grabbed me and gave me a big hug.

It was a wonderful moment. I have never been more proud of being the author of *Mosby's Tour Guide to Nursing School*. Over the years this book has helped many people—men and women—get through nursing school, and it can help you, too.

First, it will help you decide if nursing is a good career choice for you. It will help you pick the right school, calculate the costs, and then find the money and other resources you need to be successful.

Here's the information you need on everything from boosting your test scores to boosting your self-esteem, from conducting a study group to overcoming procrastination, from choosing electives to improving term papers, from handling failure to conquering prejudice. Plus you will find candid comments, examples, and ideas from other nursing students.

This is the sixth edition. That means it's been around the block a few times. Everything has been updated. It's also been expanded. There is a new chapter to introduce you to state boards or NCLEX, the final to end all finals. Forewarned is forearmed. The last chapter will help you find the best possible first job as a nurse.

One outstanding feature of this survival guide is that it tackles the challenges faced by a "mature" student. Nursing educators used to call anyone older than 20 and other than female a "nontraditional" student. Today female students younger than 20 are the exception, not the rule. Although typical nursing students are still overwhelmingly female, men are also finding rewarding careers in nursing. Nursing students are older and wiser and much more encumbered than they used to be. Students bring a lot of baggage— obligations, responsibilities, commitments, constraints, and conflicts—all of which make being a successful student much more challenging.

You've picked a good time to enter nursing school. The demand for nurses has never been greater. Salaries are excellent! Scholarships, loans, and grants are readily available. Accelerated programs that take students with degrees in other fields and convert them into nurses in record time, are rapidly expanding.

Although this book was originally designed for the "first-time travelers," nurses returning for advanced degrees and experienced students from other fields making a career switch into nursing have reported the strategies and suggestions in the *Tour Guide* most helpful.

Most travelers on this route have a lot in common. Most of us are practical idealists. You know—the sort of people who want to save the human race but who also know the value of a regular paycheck. As a practical idealist myself, I know it's not easy keeping your feet on the ground while your head is in the clouds. Nursing is one of the few professions that enables you to make such a long stretch. Although you will not be able to save the whole planet, occasionally you will save one of its occupants. That will be enough.

From the beginning this book has been a collaborative effort. Not only has it involved Mosby, the National Student Nurses' Association, and me, it reflects input from countless students and nurses throughout the United States and Canada.

You are the only person who can make this book better. Your input can make sure this tour guide/survival kit keeps doing the job it was designed to do—help nursing students survive and even thrive.

If you would like to make a suggestion, share an experience, give a recommendation, or pass along a hot tip, write to me. I promise to respond.

Have a wonderful trip to nursing!

Melodie Chenevert, RN, BSN, MN, MA
c/o Nursing Division, Elsevier Inc.
3251 Riverport Lane
Maryland Heights, MO 63043

Foreword

Imagine a CareerQuest program, similar to MapQuest—just plug in the variables (destination, specialty, educational requirements, mentor selection, etc.) and like magic, a road map to your career is downloaded and available whenever you need it! Maybe this is not far in the future but in the meantime, you have this incredible *Tour Guide to Nursing School* to help you to map out your future in nursing.

Nursing school can frequently be like a labyrinth—a maze of connecting passageways leading in many directions with a multitude of possibilities for the future. One can become trapped by even just one wrong turn and it may take several turns to get back on track. Like every puzzle it is wise to have all of the pieces sorted out and at least some idea of the big picture before beginning to put the pieces together. Just imagine hovering over the labyrinth so that the path can be clearly visualized and easily mapped out.

Think of this book as your guide through the complexities of nursing school and the profession you seek to enter. Keep it at your side and refer to it often. It is written in a lighthearted easy-to-read format and no memorization is necessary. It is user friendly and a great investment of your time—read it more than once to get the full impact of the message. Each chapter will help to make your journey more enjoyable and not only will you survive nursing school—you will thrive in nursing school!

Like all puzzles the pieces eventually fall into place, and the same is true for nursing school. But you cannot complete the puzzle alone! Support and encouragement will come from many sources helping you make your way successfully out of the labyrinth into the world of professional nursing. *Mosby's Tour Guide to Nursing School* is your CareerQuest to get you from here to there—enjoy the journey!

Diane J. Mancino, EdD, RN, CAE
Executive Director, National Student Nurses' Association
www.nsna.org

Contents

MOSBY'S
TOUR GUIDE TO
NURSING SCHOOL

A Student's Road Survival Kit

In collaboration with NSNA
National Student Nurses' Association, Inc.

CHAPTER 1

Ticket to Ride

"Finding meaningful, absorbing work is one of the straightest routes to a happier life."
—ANNA QUINDLEN

Did you ever stop at a tourist information booth? There are racks full of brochures telling you everything to see and do. The sponsors of these information booths want you to enjoy your visit so much you'll want to live there.

If I were designing a brochure for nursing, it would look something like this:

Nursing

It's more than a good living. It's a good life!

Good living. The average nursing salary is about $65,000 a year. Fringe benefits are excellent. Job security is unparalleled. Because the nurse shortage is a national crisis, generous scholarships and interest-free loans are available for basic and advanced education.

Good life. Nursing is the most portable career you can have. You can get a job literally anywhere in the world. Flexible schedules make it possible to combine a fulfilling family life and a challenging career. You can work in a hospital, clinic, school, home health agency, or industry; you can join the military or create your own business. There are opportunities in education, management, and research. As a nurse you will help people of all ages, incomes, races, religions, and cultures. Yes, becoming a nurse is hard work and being a nurse is a tough job, but every day you will be someone's hero.

Then I'd tell you 101 things you could see and do. For example:

As a new nurse your first job will probably be in a hospital. You will be able to choose from dozens of opportunities. In fact, you could spend your entire career in one hospital and never explore all the options.

First, there are so many different clinical specialties. Just name any body part and there is a specialty built around it—eyes, ears, nose, toes, bones, heart, guts, brain. Then choose whether you want to be a *bedside nurse* giving direct patient care, a *specialist,* an *educator,* a *researcher,* a *supervisor,* a manager, or an *executive.* There are *admission nurses* and *discharge planning nurses* and nurses who serve as *patient advocates.* You could be an *infection control nurse* or work in quality assurance.

You might work in a physician's office or a clinic. You might choose urgent care where people who don't have a family physician but who don't need an emergency department can go for treatment. You might choose to work in an emergency department, become a *trauma nurse specialist,* or a *triage nurse* who sorts patients and prioritizes their needs. You might be the *transport nurse* in the ambulance or the *flight-for-life nurse* on a helicopter.

You might choose surgery. There are many different roles for nurses in and around the operating room. You might prepare patients for surgery; be the *scrub nurse* or *first assistant* who acts as the doctor's right hand, be a *nurse anesthetist* who puts patients to sleep and monitors them throughout surgery, or be the *postanesthesia nurse* who keeps patients safe until they are awake, alert, and transferred to a regular hospital room.

You might be a *neuroscience nurse* specializing in brain tumors, strokes, or spinal cord injuries. You can provide care when patients are gravely ill or when they are in rehabilitation re-learning the basics such as how to walk, talk, read, or eat.

If you like cutting-edge technology, you can work as a *critical care nurse.* You can be a nurse on the *transplant team,* transplanting hearts, lungs, livers, kidneys, bone marrow, and more. *Dialysis nurses* work with patients who are waiting for kidney transplants or who are ineligible for transplants. Oncology nurses work with cancer patients. Some become chemotherapy or radiation therapy experts.

Do you like babies? Then you might work in labor and delivery or the newborn nursery. You can teach prenatal classes for expectant moms and dads. You could become a *nurse-midwife* and deliver babies in homes as well as in hospitals. (Nurse-midwives in rural areas used to ride horseback. You'll be glad to know that today they drive cars.) You might be a *well-baby nurse specialist* or a *neonatal intensive care unit (NICU) nurse* helping the tiniest babies survive and thrive. You can be a *lactation consultant,* helping mothers be successful at breastfeeding. There are nurse sonographers who do ultrasound tests to monitor unborn babies and nurses who specialize in *genetic counseling.*

At the other end of the spectrum are *hospice nurses* who help patients and their families in the last stages of life have a dignified, comfortable death. Palliative care nurses provide comfort to patients undergoing difficult treatments. They specialize in pain management and symptom control.

Variety is the spice of life for *medical-surgical* nurses. They care for patients in every category. Orthopedic nurses specialize in treating patients with bone and joint injuries and disorders. *Cardiac nurses* work with heart patients in all phases of their care. You can work in the burn unit.

Gerontology nurses care for the oldest old. *Pediatric nurses* care for children through adolescence. Both do everything a general medical-surgical nurse would do but with a twist. The very young and the very old have special needs during surgery, acute care, and rehabilitation.

You can be a *camp nurse* for kids or run an *adult daycare* center for older adults. You can work in a *nursing home.* You can own a nursing home!

You could become a public health nurse and work in the community. You might be a *visiting nurse* who sees people in their homes. You might specialize in the needs of migrant workers, join the Indian Health Service, or work with the homeless. You could be a *Peace Corps volunteer,* sign on with the World Health Organization (WHO), or serve on the *Ship Hope* as it sails the world providing state-of-the-art care to underserved populations. You could become a *cruise ship nurse* and care for the idle rich. Club Med and Disneyland hire nurses too!

You might become a *medical missionary* and travel to the remote corners of the earth. Or you could become a *parish nurse,* sponsored by your local church to care for its parishioners and reach out to those in need right in your own neighborhood.

If you have an itch to travel, you can sign up with a *traveling nurse* agency. These agencies usually place nurses for 3- to 6-month assignments. All expenses are paid, and traveling nurses may earn twice as much as regular nurses.

School nurses work with students in preschool programs right up through college health clinics. They do some first aid, lots of health screening and physical exams, and even more teaching, counseling, and consulting.

As a *research nurse,* you could work at any university. You might go to Washington, D.C., and work at the National Institutes of Health (NIH), where nurses are doing procedures that are too new or too intensive for a general hospital or that require much more laboratory and scientific support than it could provide. Or you might go to Atlanta and work for the Centers for Disease Control and Prevention (CDC). You might become a *clinical trials project manager* who sets timelines, tracks projects, develops budgets, and secures contracts. You could become a *drug safety* monitor.

You might work for an insurance company doing health screening and physical exams. You can decide which procedures are covered by the policy and whether or not to reimburse hospitals and physicians. You might be an *investigator* and look for fraud.

You might be a *legal nurse consultant* and serve as an expert witness in trials. You can become a *nurse attorney.* You can become a *Sexual Assault*

Nurse Examiner (SANE) who examines rape victims, preserves evidence, acts as an advocate, and provides counseling. Nurses also work in prisons and other correctional facilities.

Nurses serve in the military. Where there are troops or battlefields, you will always find nurses. You might work in a veterans hospital or even become a *four-star general!*

The *health and fitness* industry hires lots of nurses to help folks do everything from lose weight to stop smoking. *Occupational health nurses* work for small businesses and large corporations. (Healthy employees mean a healthy bottom line.) They do lots of troubleshooting and preventive health care. They provide employee-assistance programs to help people in crisis or people with addictions.

You can work as a *psychiatric nurse,* helping everyone from autistic children to elders with Alzheimer's disease. You can be a *therapist in private practice* seeing patients independently or you can work for a mental health clinic, group home, or state hospital. You can answer crisis hotline calls, deal with suicide prevention, or become a stress management specialist.

Teaching is part of every nurse's job, but some nurses specialize in teaching. *Inservice educators* keep the staff informed about new policies, procedures, medications, and equipment. *Patient educators* teach patients and their families about their illnesses, medications, treatments, and options. Schools of nursing have *deans, professors, assistant professors, instructors, teaching assistants, research assistants, guest lecturers,* and *clinical faculty.* Clinically speaking, you might become a diabetes educator or an asthma expert.

You could become a *case manager* who coordinates care for patients with chronic illnesses, making sure treatment is not overdone or left undone.

Clinical nurse specialists are usually experts in one clinical area (heart, lung, maternal-child, cancer). They teach other health care professionals how to give optimum care. They also provide direct care to patients and families as well as coordinate multidisciplinary teams.

Nurse practitioners are supercharged nurses who often substitute for physicians as primary caregivers, perform advanced procedures, and prescribe drugs.

Pharmaceutical companies and hospital equipment manufacturers love to hire nurses as *sales representatives.* Nurses become *consultants* to architectural firms, human resource companies, the motion picture industry, and politicians. Nurses become *politicians!* Nurses have been elected to the House and the Senate.

Nurses become *authors* and *editors.* Nurses become *inventors* and *entrepreneurs.* There are *nurse ethicists, nurse sociologists,* and *nurse anthropologists.* And the list goes on.

It's been said that the average person will have three careers and 6 to 10 jobs in a lifetime. If you become a nurse, you can do that and never leave nursing!

Some of these options require advanced degrees or additional licenses. But many of these just require guts, gumption, persistence, and imagination.

But before you can explore any of these opportunities, you need to go to nursing school. It's your ticket to the ride of a lifetime.

CHAPTER 2

The Starting Lineup

"Nothing great was ever achieved without enthusiasm."
—RALPH WALDO EMERSON

The first thing many students do is size up the competition. They think of getting an education as a fiercely competitive race. They jockey for first position as though only one student will be allowed to graduate.

Whether or not you're this competitive, it's only human to look at your classmates and wonder about your comparative status. You may even begin to wonder whether the faculty knew what they were doing when they admitted you. After all, how can they expect you to compete with a fellow who served as a medic in the military, a woman who is old enough to be your mother, a high school valedictorian, and a person who holds a bachelor's degree in psychology?

Relax. You are not expected to compete with other students. You are expected to cooperate with them.

Instead of a race, think of this educational venture as a caravan about to undertake a long journey. The ultimate goal is to get everyone in your class to the final destination. It is cooperation, not competition, that will bring you success.

Everyone in your class has an excellent chance to graduate because everyone here is already a winner. All have won a place at the starting gate. Considering the rigors of the admission process: getting here was no small accomplishment. If you have managed to get admitted to a school of nursing, YOU CAN DO ANYTHING!

So start your engines. We're off and running.

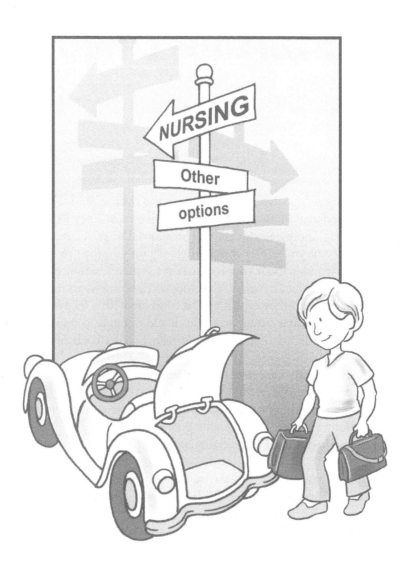

CHAPTER 3

Is This Trip Really Necessary?

"I shall be telling this with a sigh
Somewhere ages and ages hence:
Two roads diverged in a wood,
and I—I took the one less traveled by,
And that has made all the difference."
—ROBERT FROST, "The Road Not Taken"

Before you follow the yellow brick road to nursing, double-check to make sure you know where you are going and what you will find when you get there. Be sure to separate fact from fantasy. For example, if you think a nurse's primary function is to assist a physician, you have been watching too much television. In real life nurses spend very little time working alongside physicians. Nurses usually work alone.

What Do Nurses Do All Day?

Nursing is not a do-as-you-are-told job. It is a profession that demands the ability to interview, observe, analyze, detect, develop, write, teach, interpret, counsel, coordinate, collaborate, insert, inject, dispense, change, document, count, order, improvise, supervise, create, give, and take.

In one day you may be called on to do such diverse tasks as interview patients, document progress, develop care plans, write discharge summaries, teach self-care, interpret laboratory findings, insert tubes, check monitors, maintain life-support machinery, counsel grief-stricken families, collaborate with other health care professionals, analyze problems, assess potentials, irrigate wounds, change dressings, collect specimens, coordinate care during birth or death, dispense medications, take temperatures, and give hope.

Much of a nurse's time is spent in direct patient care. Most nurses wish it could be more. Unfortunately, nurses are also saddled with lots of other tasks, such as transcribing physicians' orders, counting narcotics, ordering supplies, directing traffic, enforcing policies, maintaining schedules, answering telephones, delivering dinner trays, cleaning utility rooms, obtaining equipment, running errands, and mopping up messes.

The general-duty, all-purpose, industrial-strength registered nurse must be ready, willing, and able to deliver everything from mail to babies. Obviously it takes much more than a nice personality, a ready smile, and good intentions to make a good nurse. It takes more substance than fluff to be a successful nurse.

Are you fluff or substance? To find out, take this quiz:

DO YOU HAVE...

1.	A strong background in math and science?	☐ Yes	☐ No
2.	Good hand-eye coordination?	☐ Yes	☐ No
3.	Lots of common sense?	☐ Yes	☐ No
4.	The ability to stay calm in emergencies?	☐ Yes	☐ No
5.	Excellent communication skills?	☐ Yes	☐ No
6.	A sound body?	☐ Yes	☐ No
7.	A stable mind?	☐ Yes	☐ No
8.	An above-average intellect?	☐ Yes	☐ No
9.	An affinity for machines and computers?	☐ Yes	☐ No
10.	A compassionate heart?	☐ Yes	☐ No
11.	Teaching abilities?	☐ Yes	☐ No
12.	Leadership qualities?	☐ Yes	☐ No
13.	Patience, tolerance, flexibility, persistence?	☐ Yes	☐ No
14.	A strong ego?	☐ Yes	☐ No
15.	An affinity for problem solving?	☐ Yes	☐ No
16.	Confidence in your decision-making abilities?	☐ Yes	☐ No
17.	Good organizational skills?	☐ Yes	☐ No
18.	Reliable powers of observation?	☐ Yes	☐ No
19.	The ability to see the best in people in the worst of times?	☐ Yes	☐ No
20.	No objection to working on Christmas?	☐ Yes	☐ No

FILL IN ONE BLOCK FOR EVERY "YES" ANSWER

FLUFF   **SUBSTANCE**
☐ ☐ ☐ ☐ ☐ ☐ ☐ ☐ ☐ ☐ ☐ ☐ ☐ ☐ ☐ ☐ ☐ ☐ ☐ ☐

If you have all the qualities outlined in the quiz, skip nursing and go directly to sainthood. You are not only too good for nursing, you are too good to be true. But the more of these attributes you have, the more likely you are to make a success of nursing—and the more likely nursing is to make a success of you.

What Nursing is and What it Isn't

If you think nursing is an insurance policy—something nice to "fall back on" in case you are forced to work outside the home at some point in the future— think again. Rapid developments in science and technology make it difficult even for working nurses to keep their skills current.

Nurses who drop out of the profession for a few years have found it increasingly difficult, and sometimes impossible, to reenter nursing. The once-a-nurse-always-a-nurse guarantee may have expired. For example, a nurse who had been out of the profession for 10 years decided to return to nursing. At every interview she was told that first choice in hiring went to employed nurses seeking transfers, second choice went to new graduates, and third choice went to former nurses who had completed a refresher course. The Catch-22 was that there were no refresher courses being offered in her state at that time.

If you think nursing is the road to perpetual job security, think again. For more than 40 years that was essentially true because the demand for nurses exceeded the supply. By 1984, however, astonished nurses in many parts of the United States suddenly faced layoffs and a very tight job market.

Although analysts saw this surplus of nurses as an artificial glitch and predicted the shortage would soon reappear, the damage was already done. Potential nursing students turned away from the profession in droves. In 1986 schools of nursing reported drops in enrollment of up to 50%.

That bad news soon proved to be good news for nurses and nursing students. As the economy recovered, the demand for nurses skyrocketed. Funding for education increased. Salaries shot up dramatically. Hospitals went to great lengths to attract and keep good nurses.

The nurse shortage made national headlines. Schools of nurses were filled to overflowing. In 1993, for every student admitted to a school of nursing, two students had to be turned away.

But by then the nation's economy was in serious trouble. The early 1990s looked just like the early 1980s. The nurse shortage? What nurse shortage? Hospitals were merging, downsizing, and closing. Suddenly, experienced nurses flooded the market. In many areas of the country, new graduates were hard pressed to find entry-level positions.

Boom. Bust. Boom. Bust.

In the late 1990s, hospitals continued to "dispose" of nurses, hoping to replace them with less expensive personnel. Salaries stagnated, fringe benefits were reduced, and important perks such as flexible schedules disappeared. Nurses entered the new millennium battered and bruised.

Overnight something changed. Suddenly hospitals were bulging with patients, and there weren't enough nurses to provide care. Actually, it wasn't sudden at all. Our population is aging, and older people just require more care.

Hospitals that had pitched out nurses were now asking their nurses to pitch in—to work double shifts, come in on their days off, and cancel vacations. But the nurses had aged, too. Many were not ready, willing, or able to rise to the challenge.

In 2001 the nurse shortage was again a national crisis. Déjà vu. Enrollment in schools of nursing had declined steadily over the previous 6 years. In one prestigious school of nursing, the number of freshmen entering had dropped from 90 to 25.

Local, state, and federal task forces began working frantically to reverse the trend. Money was pumped into scholarships and interest-free loans. Nurse recruiters, used to attending high school career fairs, found themselves promoting nursing in middle schools, elementary schools, and even preschools!

Johnson & Johnson pumped millions of dollars into a public service advertising campaign to promote nursing as great career. You have probably seen their television ads. If you haven't visited their website, you should. It is www.discovernursing.com.

At the dawn of 2009 with the global economy in shambles and staggering unemployment rates, nursing looked great. The U.S. Bureau of Labor Statistics was projecting a need for a million new and replacement registered nurses by 2016. But by May 2009 there were hiring freezes in many hospitals, and newly minted nurses were entering a tough job market.

Sound familiar?

Whenever the economy stumbles, nurses who work part-time ask to work full-time, and older nurses delay retirement. That is precisely because *nurses have the most reliable income of any family member.*

If you are lucky, you will be in school during the "bust" and graduate just in time for the "boom."

Health care reform is on the way, but what that reform will actually entail is anyone's guess. Because nursing is the largest health care profession, with approximately 3 million members, it promises to be an exciting time for us.

Today almost 60% of all nurses work in hospitals. The rest work in other settings—home, school, clinic, community. You will hear a lot about advanced practice nurses. These are nurses with graduate degrees who are equipped to provide primary care.

People who choose nursing usually have other interests besides just making a living. They are looking for a way of life that is compatible with their humanitarian instincts.

Having a relative or a friend with a severe handicap or health problem can be a real source of inspiration. It can also be a real source of guilt.

Will you be successful and happy as a nurse? Yes, if you are reliable, responsible, adaptable, studious, curious, tolerant, generous, discreet, and in good physical and emotional health. Having a sense of humor is also important according to a two-page advertisement from the New York Life Insurance Company published in the *Saturday Evening Post* back in 1955. I happened upon it in an antique store.

New York Life had sponsored a series of advertisements on career opportunities ranging from farming to teaching to engineering. The series was designed to help parents assess which careers might be right for their children.

At the end of the piece, it said that if you "have the qualities of mind and heart and spirit that nursing demands" you will receive, "in return, rewards far beyond wealth—rewards that never can be lost or stolen: a life of stimulating contacts, honor and respect in your community, and the priceless satisfaction of knowing that every hour of your working life has been of use to others."

That's still true.

CHAPTER **4**

Destination:
Registered Nurse

Being a Nurse Means...

You will never be bored.
You will always be frustrated.
You will be surrounded by challenges—so much to do and so little time.
You will carry immense responsibility with very little authority.
You will step into people's lives, and you will make a difference.
Some will bless you. Some will curse you.
You will see people at their worst—and at their best. You will never cease to be
*   amazed at people's capacity for love, courage, and endurance.*
You will see life begin and end.
You will experience resounding triumphs and devastating failures.
You will cry a lot.
You will laugh a lot.
You will know what it is to be human and to be humane.
—MELODIE CHENEVERT

Welcome to nursing! It is the most exasperating career ever invented. It is also the most fulfilling.

Although I've written several books for nurses, the most popular piece I have written is that poem. It is often read at pinning ceremonies and graduations.

If you choose to become a nurse, I can guarantee you intangible rewards that can rarely be matched by any other profession.

Here's more good news: The tangible rewards for being a nurse are also excellent.

At the start of 2009, the average nurse, working full-time in an acute care setting, was making about $65,000 a year. Starting salaries averaged between $37,000 and $52,000 a year, depending primarily on geographic area. Inexperienced nurses made from $21 to $27 per hour; experienced nurses, $28 to $59 per hour, and some highly specialized nurses topped $150 per hour.

As you investigate salaries, it may appear that there are some significant variations around the country. However, if you adjust those salaries in terms of cost of living, the differences effectively evaporate. For example, it costs twice as much to live half as well in New York City as it does in rural Georgia.

What other tangible rewards can you expect from nursing? The quickest way is to look at the most current career opportunity guides published annually by nursing journal companies. Hospitals spend big bucks advertising in these guides, hoping to entice nurses to come work for them.

Nursing Career Guide Decoder Kit

In the 2009 career guides, these were some of the perquisites hospitals were proud to offer:

- Free family hospitalization plan
- College scholarships for your children
- Household goods moved and billed directly to the hospital
- $3000 bonus after first 30 days
- 24-hour onsite child care
- Relocation allowance up to $12,000
- 37.5-hour workweek
- 13 holidays per year
- 3 weeks of vacation—the first year!
- Half of all weekends off
- No state income tax
- Physical fitness center and pool
- Tuition reimbursement for senior year
- Up to $8000 for student loan forgiveness
- Tuition reimbursement up to $7500 per semester for advanced degree
- NO SHIFT ROTATION
- Uniform allowance
- Loyalty bonus up to $2500
- Weekend bonus of 25%
- Free parking
- Quality preceptorships
- Base pay up to $42 per hour

- 401(k) plan
- Health, dental, and vision coverage from day one
- Discounts on prescription drugs
- Discount mortgages and home equity loans
- Tax-sheltered annuities
- Evening/night differentials (ranging from less than $3000 to more than $12,000 per year)

Read between the lines. This is the good stuff. These hospitals are boasting. That means a lot of hospitals offer less vacation, fewer holidays, no tuition reimbursement, no uniform allowance, no bonuses for weekend work, no dental insurance, and little differential for working evenings or nights. It also means that many hospitals will require you to rotate shifts and to work more than half of the weekends.

You are not stupid. You know sick people need care around the clock, 7 days a week, 365 days a year, including weekends and holidays. However, you might not have considered what that would mean to you as a working nurse.

One hospital stated in its ad that "mandatory overtime" had been eliminated for nurses with 5 years of service. That means if you have been with the hospital for less than 5 years, you will be required to work overtime.

Some hospitals are offering incentives such as job sharing, flexible schedules, sick child care, spa memberships, free maid service, and even sign-on bonuses of cold, hard cash. In fact, the Army was advertising a $20,000 to $30,000 sign-on bonus, or you could choose a $10,000 sign-on bonus plus up to $120,000 to repay your education loans!

There has been increasing emphasis on retaining nurses, not just recruiting them. Many hospitals have discontinued sign-on bonuses in favor of retention bonuses and other incentives for loyal nurses. Here are some examples:

- Comprehensive orientation with one-on-one preceptors
- E-learning center with 24-hour access
- Pristine state-of-the-art facilities
- Great patient/nurse ratio
- The flexibility you need to balance career and family time
- Domestic partner insurance
- Generous commitment incentives
- Concierge services
- On-site BSN and MSN programs
- Fellowships and internships
- Shared governance (a management philosophy in which nurses are respected, included in decision making, and have control over their practice)

Nursing continues to provide better-than-average benefits for its full-time and part-time workers in important areas such as health insurance, pension plans, sick days, and vacations than most other industries.

Compressed salary scales are less of a problem than they used to be. Not long ago salary differences for inexperienced and experienced nurses varied as little as 10% to 15%. Today there is a 30% to 50% difference.

What will nursing be like by the time you graduate? There's only one way to find out. Come along for the ride.

CHAPTER 5

How Long Will This Trip Take?

"The cost of a thing is the amount of what I call life which is required to be exchanged for it, immediately, or in the long run."
—HENRY DAVID THOREAU

When you first learned that there are three different routes (associate degree, diploma, baccalaureate) to becoming a registered nurse, you may have decided to take the fastest, cheapest, most convenient route. After all, who in his or her right mind would spend twice as much time and money to end up with the same credential? A nurse is a nurse.

That is like saying a car is a car. Although the statement is essentially true, it is not the whole truth. For example, a Volkswagen and a Mercedes are fine automobiles. Either will provide you with years of dependable transportation. The Mercedes, however, comes equipped with many options not available on the Volkswagen.

If you are enrolled in an associate degree or diploma program, you will emerge driving an economy car. Good job opportunities will be available to you, but many career opportunities will be inaccessible unless you "trade up." Some hospitals make little monetary distinction between nurses with and nurses without a bachelor's degree. However, those same hospitals often refuse to promote a staff nurse who lacks a BSN degree.

The debate over educational preparation for nurses has raged for five decades and is hotly contested. It is perhaps the most divisive and potentially destructive issue facing nursing.

I have been a student in two of the three programs and a teacher in all of them. I would be the first to tell you that the length of the program is no guarantee of quality. Admirable programs and abominable programs exist at every level. It is all in the engineering.

When you look for a nursing program, make sure you pick one that is "accredited" by the state and meets national nursing school standards. If you don't, you may lose a lot of time and money.

After you finish your education, you will be required to complete a comprehensive set of exams to secure licensure as a registered nurse. To find how well your prospective nursing school is engineered, ask about its failure rates on state board examinations for the past 5 years. Not long ago a 5% failure rate meant "heads would roll"; the dean or director would be called on the carpet. Now the average failure rate is closer to 20%. Again, length of the program is not a factor. There are 2-year programs with a 0% failure rate and 4-year programs with a 37% failure rate. Make sure you go with a winner, or your trip could take much longer than expected. In fact, you might never arrive!

Looking Beyond the Horizon

It is not a question of becoming a nurse. All three paths lead to nursing. The question is, what do you want to do after you become a nurse? What sort of job would you like to have 5 years after graduation? Ten years after graduation?

At this stage of your journey, projecting yourself that far into the future may be nigh unto impossible. Just becoming a nurse seems light years away. All you want to do is get that RN behind your name and get a job. Graduating from any nursing school will open the door to an excellent job. But some of you want a lot more than a job. Some of you already have very definite ideas of where you want to go once you become a nurse.

If you envision yourself as a public health nurse, clinical specialist, nurse practitioner, researcher, consultant, teacher, manager, or vice president of patient services, you will need a bachelor's degree at the very least. Yes, the price of a baccalaureate education is high, but the cost of not having one may be even higher.

For most career-oriented nurses, a bachelor's degree is only the beginning. Many find that their chosen destination in nursing requires a trip to graduate school.

Our profession has lagged behind others in standardizing its educational requirements. Think about physical therapists, occupational therapists, dietitians, pharmacists, and social workers. All require a bachelor's degree as minimal preparation, and many require a master's degree or above before full professional privileges are granted. For physicians, a bachelor's degree is required before they are even eligible for entrance into their professional school. Nursing has some catching up to do.

What happens if you get an associate's degree in nursing or are a diploma graduate and somewhere down the road you decide you want more options? You take your "vehicle" back to the "factory" (college or university). Many colleges are purists. They will insist you cannot have a Mercedes chassis powered by a Volkswagen engine. They will offer to rebuild your vehicle completely if you can come up with enough money and approximately 3 more years of your life. Other colleges act more like body shops. They will be happy to customize your vehicle for less time and money.

Few students receive adequate counseling before they choose a school of nursing. They often learn about the advantages and disadvantages of their particular program in their last semester.

Older students with jobs and families may find the local community college is essentially the only choice they have if they want to become a nurse. Unfortunately, only about 15% of Associate Degree Nurse (ADN) graduates go on to obtain their BSN degree and of those only about 4% obtain a graduate degree.

Studies, especially those from the University of Pennsylvania led by Linda Aiken, have demonstrated that the better educated the nurse, the better the patient outcomes. Put simply, the more baccalaureate-prepared nurses on the staff, the more patients stayed alive. This has spurred new interest in having a better educated nursing workforce. New York and New Jersey have introduced legislation that would require ADN nurses to obtain their BSN degree within 10 years. Failure to do so would mean losing their license to practice. Other state nursing associations including Colorado, Kentucky, North Carolina, and Washington are supporting this movement.

According to the *Community College Journal* (February/March 2009) this is known as "degree creep." There is concern that not only nursing but also respiratory therapy and physician assistant programs will pull out of the community college system. That would mean an enormous loss of revenue. But it doesn't have to be an either/or situation. It can be an either/and situation.

Oregon Health Sciences University (OHSU) School of Nursing is a stellar example of how associate degree and baccalaureate programs can cooperate instead of compete. Six Oregon community colleges have a unique partnership with OHSU. Completing the associate's degree means the students have already completed 75% of the requirements for a BSN degree. Then OHSU allows students in good standing to be automatically enrolled in the university for their 400-level nursing courses. Student loans can be continued through dual enrollment. Scholarships and financial aid are available. Classes are offered online, at their local community colleges, and at appropriate clinical sites.

This groundbreaking program is a win-win situation for nurses, colleges, and, most importantly, for patients.

Accelerate to Warp Speed

Students who already have a baccalaureate degree in another field don't have to start over from scratch to become nurses. Accelerated programs for "second-degree" students generally take 12 to 18 months to get a BSN or about 3 years to get a master's degree in nursing.

There are at least 300 accelerated BSN and master's programs. All require backbreaking course loads and intensely challenging clinical experiences. Many find the nursing degree more difficult than their first degree but these are highly motivated, mature students who have a proven track record. They are academically strong, active in student and professional organizations, and almost invariably pass state board exams on the first try.

Although the accelerated programs are expensive, hospitals love these graduates and often fully fund their education in return for a specified work commitment. Employers say it saves them a lot in recruitment costs and guarantees them outstanding employees.

Check it Out

Check the backgrounds and credentials of your instructors and the nurses you come to admire. You will find most of them have been in and out of school customizing their "vehicles" many times. You will see that your basic preparation will not determine how far you can go in nursing, but it will affect the amount of time it takes to get there.

Think carefully about the options you want and what you can "afford," not just in terms of dollars but also in terms of time and distance.

CHAPTER **6**

How Much Will This Trip Cost?

"Look at me: I worked my way up from nothing to a state of extreme poverty."
—Groucho Marx, *Monkey Business*

Before starting any trip, it is wise to estimate the costs. Otherwise you may end up stranded and not only penniless, but also deep in debt.

There are more than 1500 nursing programs in the United States. The cost can range from less than $3500 a year at a community college to more than $45,000 a year at a private college. These costs reflect tuition only. They do not include room and board and such miscellaneous expenses as books, uniforms, special equipment, travel, and laboratory fees. Books, for example, average almost $750 per year. (Your first-year book bill may be significantly higher because many of the books required in the freshman year are used throughout the entire program.)

When estimating costs, don't forget to include such incidentals as transportation to and from the clinical area, babysitters, and eating on the run.

One major cost often overlooked is that of deferred income—money you would have made if you had worked instead of going to school. If you allow $20,000 per year (a salary of $10 per hour), you can quickly see that the cost of not working will be $40,000 or $60,000 or $80,000, depending on whether you are enrolled in an associate degree, diploma, or baccalaureate program.

How much will your trip to nursing cost? Sit down with your classmates and discuss all the potential costs, including deferred income. Work through the following exercise. The total figure will be quite a jolt.

Of course there are ways to defray costs. You may be eligible for a scholarship, grant, or loan. Scholarships are usually given for academic achievement, whereas grants are based strictly on financial need. Student loans tend to carry very low interest charges, and repayment is not required until after graduation. Unlike loans, scholarships and grants do not have to be repaid.

Cost estimates of spending _____ years at _____ school of nursing	
Tuition	_____
Room and board	_____
Books	_____
Uniforms/special equipment	_____
Laboratory fees	_____
Transportation	_____
Deferred income	_____
Other:	
_____	_____
_____	_____
_____	_____
TOTAL	_____

Megabucks in Motion

To find money to help finance your education, start with Johnson & Johnson's website www.discovernursing.com. I grew up in Iowa so I thought it would be fun to see what nursing programs are available there. The website found 33 programs and 272 scholarships. It gave me basic statistics about each one and listed their websites, and had a hot button to "Find scholarships to match this program."

When it comes to finding money, don't be shy. Ask local hospitals, auxiliaries, nursing associations, service clubs, and fraternal orders about their scholarship programs. Check the public library. Even if you are 40 years old, call your local high school counselor for advice. Don't forget the armed forces. They have some excellent scholarship and financial aid benefits. Valuable information also may be obtained by contacting the National League for Nursing, the American Nurses Association (ANA), your state chapter of the ANA, the National Student Nurses' Association, and the Canadian Nurses Association. (Addresses can be found in Appendixes B, C, and D.) In 2009 *Minority Nurse* listed almost 100 scholarship sources for minority students.

Monies are available from the public as well as the private sectors. Because eligibility requirements and dollar amounts change annually, your best source of current information will be the financial aid office at your nursing school. You may also be eligible for a work-study program. Remember, just because you didn't start with a scholarship, grant, or loan doesn't mean you can't get one. Some monies become available only after you complete lower-division courses. Appendix B contains addresses you need to find out more about undergraduate financial aid and student loan programs.

Nursing students have taken out second mortgages, borrowed against insurance policies, and sold their boats, cars, and motorcycles to finance their education. A middle-aged student obtained a loan from her mother because "Mom always wanted me to become a nurse and she thought it was better late than never!" Another student said she was in school on "found" money. Once she decided to go to school, she found there were a lot of things she could do without.

How would you like to go to nursing school for free? Not only that, how would you like to be guaranteed a job with a great starting salary and fringe benefits? When a hospital in Pennsylvania made that offer, 48 students immediately signed up for the program. Many hospitals will pay off student loans or reimburse tuition expenses if you will agree to work there for a year or two.

At a national nursing convention I had a great conversation with a 40-something nurse. The next day she brought her 20-something daughter, also a nurse, to meet me.

I congratulated her on recruiting her daughter into our profession. "Oh, no," they said in unison. The mother hadn't recruited the daughter. The daughter had recruited the mother. Thinking her mom would be a great nurse, she offered to pay mom's tuition. And, if mom made a B average, she didn't have to pay her daughter back!

Most of you are comparison shoppers. You try to get top value for each dollar spent. You watch for sales, clip coupons, and drive miles out of the way to save a few bucks.

When it comes to educational dollars, however, some students behave in a most irrational manner. They would never dream of going to the store and asking the clerk, "What's the least I can get for 20 bucks?" Yet they plunk their tuition money down and then ask the instructor, "What's the least I can get for this and still graduate?" They concentrate on the minimum requirements instead of reaching for the maximum.

Regardless of what financial aid you manage to muster, this educational experience is still going to cost you thousands and thousands of dollars. So approach education in a business-like manner. You have "contracted" with the school for certain services. Make sure it delivers. You have "hired" these instructors. Be sure to get what you have paid for by learning and experiencing everything you can.

Be a smart consumer. Get your money's worth.

The cost of a nursing education cannot be measured in dollars alone. Another price will be paid in blood, sweat, and tears.

Now They Know

I asked students attending a National Student Nurses' Association convention to share one thing they wish they had known before deciding to major in nursing. Here are some of their answers:

"One Thing I Wish I Had Known Before I Chose to Major in Nursing Is:

...how difficult it was going to be!"

...how much reading there is."

...how much paperwork there is to do!"

...that so much outside work was required."

...that even though I was an honor student in high school, college is totally different."

...how much actual work it requires! (Or maybe I'm glad I didn't know. I might not have finished.)"

...that I would need to keep white underwear in stock for the rest of my life."

...how to prepare for the shock and trauma of the nursing class/clinical schedule."

...that fraternities may have Hell Week but nursing has Hell Years."

...about nursing school side effects—sexual dysfunction, sleeplessness, night terrors, restlessness. Then again, maybe I'm better having not known!"

...the astonishing amount of knowledge you must gain in 4 years."

...what nursing really is."

...what nurses really do."

...more about the three different ways to become an RN."

...all about the entry into practice issue! I certainly would have appreciated the honesty."

...the expense!"

...that you are no longer an individual until you graduate—you belong to the nursing program, physically and spiritually. On graduation you develop wings and fly."

...the number of clinical options available."

...how much time I would be investing (I'm married) and how much discipline I would need (and how much weight I was going to gain!)."

...how important computers and technology are."

...that at 43 years of age I would feel so completely awkward and useless. But by the beginning of the next year, I felt empowered and smart!"

CHAPTER 7

Rules of the Road

"Each is given a bag of tools,
A shapeless mass,
A book of rules;
And each must make,
Ere life is flown,
A stumbling-block
Or a stepping-stone."
—R. L. SHARPE, "Stumbling-Block or Stepping-Stone"

All schools of nursing are similar, but no two are identical. Each has designed its own highly customized track on which you will learn how to be a nurse.

On your admission the school effectively issues you a learner's permit. If you fail to follow the rules of its road, your permit may be canceled. Therefore, knowing the rules and regulations is imperative.

So READ THE RULES. Take a deep breath and read them again. Ignorance can cost you big bucks and add months to your program. Don't be caught saying "I didn't know I had to have organic chemistry first...my incomplete would automatically convert to an F...Abnormal Psychology was only offered winter quarter...three clinical absences meant I had to repeat the course...advanced registration began last week...fees were due Monday."

Check the college catalog, the student handbook, special orientation packets, and all first-day-of-class handouts. Don't just read them; study them. Underline vital information and make notes in the margins. Highlight those things that apply to you immediately or in the near future. If you have questions, get clarification. Don't rely on the grapevine for the latest word on course requirements. Go directly to the source. Talk with the instructor involved.

These policies were not written by God, but they might as well have been. They do not reflect spur-of-the-moment decisions. They are decisions that have evolved over many years. Countless deans, directors, faculty members, students, advisory boards, and ad hoc committees have devised and revised the rules and regulations governing your school of nursing.

If the rules and regulations begin to get you down, remember that what appears to be a roadblock may actually be a guardrail placed there to keep you from plunging off a cliff.

Rules and Reasons

Schools of nursing represent a huge investment in manpower and machinery. Their programs are among the most expensive to run. They are insured to the hilt and are accountable to more governmental and professional agencies than you can imagine. They will supply you with teachers, classrooms, laboratories, disposable equipment, and not-so-disposable patients. The schools shoulder an enormous responsibility. In return, you must grant them a few eccentricities.

For example, most schools have written codes for dress and behavior. This really irks some students. They consider it an infringement on their personal rights. It is nothing personal. It is strictly professional. This may be the first time your personal freedoms collide with professional responsibilities, but it won't be the last.

Before bursting into a chorus of "I've Gotta Be Me," consider the advantages of being "me" on your own time. You can avoid all sorts of headaches and hassles if you simply agree to bathe regularly, use deodorant, wear shoes, spit out your chewing gum, or give up showing off your latest body piercing.

On the school's time, be a polished professional. On your own time, cut loose, relax, and enjoy. At first you may feel absolutely schizophrenic. Gradually, the "real" you and the "professional" you will meld and mature into a "new" you.

If you want to stay in school, CONFORM. Sure, you can fight the system. But face it, you don't have the time, energy, or cunning it takes to win. You'll just end up spinning your wheels while other students drive off with diplomas.

Instead of fighting the system, use it. When conflicts arise, take your concerns, suggestions, and grievances to the student-faculty committee responsible for such matters. Then hurry back to the business of learning. After all, your job is not to revamp this school of nursing. Your job is to graduate.

There is no such thing as a perfect school of nursing, an optimum curriculum, or an ideal textbook. But we are working on it. That is why you will find curricula constantly under construction, courses being remodeled, textbooks being switched midyear, and learning experiences that seem to appear and disappear without warning. Be sure to see your advisor regularly to be aware of any upcoming changes as well as to keep tabs on your progress.

One student inquired about a computer course labeled 108X. Although the description sounded like just what she needed, she noticed that no other course in that column had an "X" rating. She was told it denoted an experimental course that was "not quite approved." She wisely chose another course that was fully approved.

When you are handed an armload of paper listing miles of rules and regulations, it is hard to believe that all of this has been compiled to make student life less complicated. On careful examination, however, you'll find that these papers do more than outline your obligations; they safeguard your opportunities. Following the instructions makes your graduation not only a possibility but a distinct probability.

Yes, there are exceptions to every rule. But are you really that exceptional?

"This is the grave of Mike O'Day
Who died maintaining his right of way.
His right was clear, his will was strong,
But he's just as dead as if he'd been wrong."

—EPITAPH

CHAPTER **8**

Slower Traffic Keep Right

"Never mistake motion for action."
—Ernest Hemmingway

If you are just starting out on your first lap around the track, listen to some student-to-student tips for success. Students attending a National Student Nurses' Association convention were asked to share one "survival" tip they would like to pass on to beginning students.

Their suggestions can be divided into four categories: (1) take care of yourself; (2) take care of each other; (3) take one day at a time; and (4) take care of business.

Take Care of Yourself

"Wear comfortable shoes."

"Look in the mirror, take a deep breath, and smile. This is the face your patients and families see."

"Set time aside each day for yourself or your family."

"Don't spend all of your time studying."

"Make sure to take care of yourself. Don't put nursing school ahead of your own health."

"Make sure you look your best every day. The better you look, the better others will treat you."

"Take 30 minutes a week to renew yourself—garden, bike, draw, write a poem."

"Eat breakfast."

"The best advice in the world is, don't take advice from anyone. You are a unique individual and your experience in nursing school will be unique as well."

"Be involved in more activities on campus than just nursing school. It helps keep your sanity."

"As our mothers always told us, you are who you hang with! Stay with people who make you feel good about yourself—no negativity. Negativity drains the soul and the mind. Any obstacle can be overcome with an open mind and a positive attitude."

"Take dance breaks while studying. It will keep you energized and in a good mood."

"Take a fun elective."

"Study hard, but play hard, too. Make time for friends. Take walks, work out, dance, swim, play tennis—it will keep you sane."

"Science and math can be learned. Caring can't. Don't let chemistry and pharmacology intimidate you and keep you from becoming a nurse!"

"Have friends outside of the nursing department—clubs, athletics, churches. Friends who are not in nursing help you get your mind off things. They are wonderful!"

"No matter how much advice you get, it won't matter unless you take it, apply it, live with it, and most important, USE IT!"

"Life is short—so is nursing school!"

Take Care of Each Other

"Treat others as you would like to be treated."

"Once you get your head above water, always offer to help others."

"Don't compete with anyone but yourself."

"Build a support system with your fellow students."

"Work together as a class. Don't let the competitive spirit get in the way."

"Get involved early with the National Student Nurses' Association (NSNA). Networking is important."

"Join a study group. I couldn't have made it without mine."

"The steps to good nursing: RAID without the bugs! R = Read material carefully. A = Apply what was learned. I = Instruct fellow classmates who do not understand. D = Demonstrate your learning during clinical practice."

"I have adult attention deficit disorder. What works for me is a group of four or five students in which everyone reads a section of the material and that person explains the material to the group. Or compare the same information in different books and discuss it in the group until everyone understands."

"Study with friends. Try studying for 50 minutes and playing or talking for 10 minutes. Repeat. It's not much of a social life, but it's better than nothing."

"Get involved with other students. They can help you, and you can help them."

Take One Day at a Time

"Take it one day, one test, one patient at a time, and don't get discouraged."

"Don't take introductory classes too seriously. They are meant to weed out students. Hang in there until clinical. You'll love it!"

"When you first enter school, write down all your reasons for going into nursing. Keep the list where you can see it every day. It will keep you from giving up when you hit a rough patch."

"Don't worry when you feel like you are behind: You are! But so is everyone else. Don't give up!"

"Live one day at a time. Once something is done, don't worry about it. Just keep doing your best at each task."

"Make the best of any situation by adjusting your attitude."

"Please yourself—be happy meeting your own personal/professional/ academic goals."

"I was the mother of five young children when I went to nursing school. If I can do it, anyone can!"

"Looking at the overall picture can be pretty scary. Just concentrate on one assignment at a time."

Take Care of Business

"Focus on how to apply what you have learned."

"Make nursing school your first priority!"

"Take classes seriously. Start out studying hard."

"You have to know the normal to understand the abnornal."

"Maintain good study habits."

"Keep up with the reading from day one."

"Do the reading as you go along. Don't wait!"

"Take the extra time needed to do extra readings."

"Read, read, read. Study, study, study. Read some more. Study some more. Don't stop!"

"Keep up with work rather than trying to catch up!"

"You will never know it all. Just know where to look it up."

"Don't try to rush through—it's a marathon, not a sprint."

"Start a good home library to use for care plans."

"Keep your notes current."

"Review notes daily."

"Organize your time. Conserve your energy."

"No significant others—unless they are science majors!"

"Use Sunday night to plan your entire week."

"Create your own flash cards."

"Be prepared for three times more work than you ever imagined."

"Type your class notes. It will help you remember."

"Take a course in stress management."

"Don't take yourself seriously. Take your commitments seriously."

"Let everyone else worry about the politics and all the other stuff YOU CAN'T CONTROL! Stay focused on your studies and what YOU CAN CONTROL!"

"In the clinical area, volunteer to help with anything—be a 'gopher' for your nurse."

"Build up your GPA before you start taking all nursing courses."

"Learn to be happy with Cs and thrilled with Bs [especially if you were a straight-A student in high school]."

"Keep all your ducks in a row so you don't quack up!"

"Get a tutor if necessary."

"Rip out the section of the book you are currently reading, put it in a plastic folder, and put the appropriate class notes with it. It will save your back and you can read it in the bathroom!"

"Do not take too many sciences in one semester."

"Make sure you're financially stable enough to work minimal hours while in school."

"Have enough food in your freezer for a year!"

"Realize that it is impossible to work full time and be a good student. If you want to survive nursing, don't try to work full time."

"Get to know your instructors."

"Make sure your teachers know you—your name, your face—you. Not your number. It makes all the difference."

"Do what the teacher tells you to do. Don't argue; just do it! It will decrease your stress and your teacher's stress, too."

"Buy a book on nursing math and bone up ahead of time."

"Don't just memorize material. Learn how to apply it."

"Ninety percent of what you learn you teach yourself. Practice! Practice! Practice! Spend as much time as you can in the lab practicing those procedures. Role-playing works."

"When your patient tells you something like, 'This is the best place to start an IV,' LISTEN!"

"Keep your sense of humor!"

"Learn how to live without sleep."

"Don't forget to breathe."

Ready? Set? Go! Take the on ramp and don't look back. Just go slowly and stay in the right lane.

CHAPTER 9

Driving Instructors

"The mediocre teacher tells. The good teacher explains. The superior teacher demonstrates. The great teacher inspires."
—William Arthur Ward

Meet your driving instructors. These are the experts you've hired to take you over the course. Get to know them. Remember that they are people first, nurses second, and teachers third.

Get to know them as people. They are human. They are not infallible, omniscient, or omnipotent. They have their likes and dislikes, their dreams and fears, their good days and bad days, their strengths and weaknesses. They have diverse cultural, familial, religious, and geographic backgrounds. Each has a different philosophy of life.

Get to know them as nurses. Find out what attracted them to nursing in the first place, where they were educated, what their clinical specialties are, where they have worked, which professional organizations they belong to, what articles or books they have written, and what their goals are. Each has a different philosophy of nursing.

Get to know them as teachers. Find out how long they have been teaching, where else they have taught, what their favorite subject matter is, and in which clinical areas they enjoy guiding students. Some instructors see themselves as scholars and researchers. Others see themselves as catalysts, facilitators, role models, or even recruiters for the nursing profession. Each has a different philosophy of teaching.

Your goal is not to "psych out" the instructors so you can get by with learning as little as possible. Your goal is to "psych out" the instructors so you can learn as much as possible.

Choice of Instructors

By identifying instructors compatible with your needs, goals, philosophy, and style, you can make learning much easier. For example, if you prefer freedom to examine, experience, and discover information for yourself, you will suffocate under an instructor who delivers formal lectures and insists that everyone stay together in lock-step fashion. On the other hand, if you are a student who prefers a lot of structure and no surprises, you might excel under such an instructor.

If at all possible, avoid instructors with whom you are dreadfully mismatched in terms of style, philosophy, or temperament. Avoid any instructor who boasts of being a harsh grader. Always remember that your number one goal is to graduate.

Keep your eyes open for instructors who are masters of their craft, intellectually stimulating, and accessible in times of trouble. Instructors are prone to clone, so stick close to those you would like to resemble when you grow up (professionally speaking).

Most instructors hold advanced degrees and, in the course of obtaining those degrees, have become highly specialized. That is why teaching teams are so common in schools of nursing. A team of instructors picks you up at point X and delivers you to point Y, where another team of specialists takes over. It's rather like a cross between a road rally and a relay race.

One for the Road

Whenever you encounter a new set of instructors, always assume the best. "These instructors are here to help me. They sincerely want me to succeed. They will do everything they can on my behalf."

Nursing schools have been under a lot of pressure to increase enrollment. But studies indicate that stuffing more students into the school is not the most effective way to get more graduates. The most effective way is to focus on retaining current students and helping them successfully complete the program. The faculty honestly does want you to succeed.

Positive attitudes are contagious. Instructors enjoy working with students who are optimistic, courteous, cooperative, self-disciplined, responsible, respectful, and proud of the work they are doing. The more of these attributes you have, the more successful you will be.

Negative attitudes are equally contagious. If you are pessimistic, uncooperative, hesitant, or uninterested, your nonverbal behavior will give away your inner thoughts. The instructors will have an uneasy feeling about you. They will begin to question your ability, and your chances of failure will be greater.

Who lives longer: pessimists or optimists? In the 1960s the Mayo Clinic routinely gave the Minnesota Multiphasic Personality Inventory (MMPI) test to its patients. One element of the MMPI was an optimism-pessimism scale.

It seems that 15% of the test takers were optimists, 15% were pessimists, and the other 70% were somewhere in the middle.

Thirty years later someone must have been rummaging around in the files and thought it would be interesting to see if there were any correlation between optimism, pessimism, and longevity. I guess we'll never know. The researcher tried to talk with the pessimists, but they were dead.

Your relationship with your nursing instructors will mirror your relationships with authority figures in general. Think about how you relate to parents, clergy, employers, police officers, and other authorities. Do you see them as friends or foes? Are you usually agreeable or argumentative? Suspicious or trusting?

There are only two totally unreasonable nursing instructors in the entire country. Invariably, one will be employed by your school of nursing. If you think you are dealing with more than one totally unreasonable instructor, you have a problem. You are either in the wrong school, the wrong profession, or both.

Teacher/Learner/Student/Nurse

You may be surprised to learn that many of your nursing instructors are students themselves. Many are working on advanced degrees. They have to write term papers and take final exams. They have to worry about their own GPAs as well as yours.

Just as the nursing profession is moving toward standardizing its educational requirements to be on a par with other professions, nursing education is moving toward requiring the same credentials held by college professors in other departments.

Only a few years ago in many schools of nursing, a bachelor's degree was considered adequate preparation for a teaching position. Today, teaching opportunities for nurses with bachelor's degrees are few and fleeting. They may be hired to help teach in the clinical setting on a temporary basis. For most faculty members, a master's degree is required, and doctoral preparation is preferred. At many colleges and universities, master's-prepared nurses are being phased out unless they are actively working toward a doctorate.

Having to be teacher and graduate student simultaneously is only one pressure felt by nursing faculty. In addition to their teaching duties, nursing faculty are also expected to engage in research, to publish widely, to be politically active, to perform community service, and to maintain competence in their clinical areas. Try adding marriage, children, or both to all of this and you have a better understanding of why faculty members are not always as accessible or patient as you would like them to be.

"Roles" Royce

On the rocky road through nursing, your instructors will play many roles. As TOUR GUIDES they will plan the itinerary, provide maps, and staff the information booth. They will lead you through unfamiliar territory, introducing you to local customs, acting as interpreters, and making sure you don't offend the natives. Because they know what's coming around each bend, they will make sure you don't miss anything. By sharing stories and anecdotes, they weave together the past, present, and future of nursing.

As CONSTRUCTION WORKERS they pave the way so you can pass quickly and safely. They flag you around potholes and other possible pitfalls. They fill in gaps, build bridges, and lay good foundations. They know that before new structures can be built, old ones must sometimes be demolished. They help you bulldoze old attitudes, habits, prejudices, and other misinformation.

As HIGHWAY PATROL OFFICERS they police the road for your patients' protection. They not only handle emergencies and accidents but also help prevent them by enforcing rules and regulations. They make sure everyone is going in the right direction at the right speed. If you break the rules, they may let you off with a warning, or they may issue a formal citation that lands you in front of the judge.

"We judge ourselves by what we feel capable of doing, while others judge us by what we have already done."
—Henry Wadsworth Longfellow

As TRAFFIC COURT JUDGES they listen to individual cases and hear appeals. They may place you on probation, fine you, or suspend your license to learn. Not all of an instructor's tasks are pleasant, but all are necessary.

CHAPTER **10**

More Miles Per Gallon

"Genius is one percent inspiration and ninety-nine percent perspiration."
—THOMAS EDISON

Think of the hours in your week as gallons of gas in your tank. Every student has precisely the same amount, yet some get much farther on their weekly tank of gas than others.

If you want to get more miles per gallon, there are two things you must do. You must learn to be more EFFICIENT and more EFFECTIVE. Being more efficient means learning to do things right. Being more effective means learning to do the right things.

When it comes to efficiency, you can get more mileage by improving your reading and writing skills than any other way. Do whatever is necessary to increase your proficiency (see "Reading and Remembering" in Chapter 13). These skills will not only bring success to you as a student, they will also give you the leading edge as a professional in years to come.

Front-running students know how to conserve fuel. They know that the difference between studying for short periods and studying for long periods is like the difference between city and highway driving. They know they will accomplish more, faster, and with less wear and tear on their machinery if they take studying up to cruising speed and hold it there for an hour, or two, or three.

But no matter how efficient you become, you still will not get where you want to go if you drive off in the wrong direction. That is where effectiveness comes into play. You not only need to read well, you need to read right—the right books, the right chapters, the right journals. You may be a faster writer and technically flawless yet write wrong—the wrong topics, the wrong themes, the wrong conclusions.

How do you know what's right and what's wrong? Ask your instructor. Listen carefully.

Improving Your Fuel Efficiency

Another way students manage to get more miles to the gallon is by driving economy models. They operate under a principle described by an ancient Italian economist named Pareto. His 80/20 principle, loosely translated, says that 80% of the value or satisfaction will come from 20% of the tasks or activities.

So if you have 10 things to do today, 2 of them will account for 80% of the day's success. Leading students are able to look at their to-do lists and zero in on the two or three activities that have the highest payoff potential. They tackle those first. If there is time left, they take care of some of the remaining items.

Floundering students make no distinction regarding the payoff value of items on their to-do lists. They begin anywhere, usually with the easiest items. By the end of the day they have accomplished 8 of the 10 items on their list. Unfortunately, they did the 8 that gave them only a 20% return on their time.

Using this proportional approach when setting priorities has some very practical applications. For example, if your instructor is a specialist in the subject matter, 80% of the test will come from lecture and only 20% will come from the readings. However, if the instructor is a specialist in cardiac care but has to pinch-hit in a psychiatric nursing course, 80% of the test will come from the readings and only 20% will come from lecture.

Once you become aware of the 80/20 principle, you will begin to see all sorts of other applications. You will notice that 80% of your homework comes from 20% of your teachers, that 80% of all prescriptions involve only 20% of the drugs, and that 80% of what you need to know is contained in 20% of your textbook. Ah…if only you knew which 20%!

Superstudents have developed the ability to pick out the 20% of the reading that gives them 80% of what they need to know. They don't try to master everything in the textbook. They concentrate on that small percentage that allows them to sail through exams and to perform competently in the clinical area. If you need help developing this ability, see Chapter 13, "Drive-Up Teller."

Here are some other tips to help you get more miles per gallon.

Time Management from A to Z for Nursing Students

Attendance. Every hour you spend in class will save you 3 hours of study time. If you are going to cut corners somewhere, go to class and skimp on study time. Attend every class.

Budgeting. Most students claim they just don't have enough time. Yet every student has all the time there is: 168 hours per week, no more and no less. Therefore, managing your time becomes even more important than managing your money because once time is spent, you can't earn more.

To make sure you use each day to the maximum, buy a pocket-sized daily planner or an electronic personal digital assistant (PDA) and keep it with you. If necessary, buy a jumbo calendar to keep track of major events. Scope the whole term, marking out such milestones as exams, term papers, and research projects. Block out all clinical times. Don't forget to allow time for preclinical work such as reading charts, making care plans, and interviewing patients.

Approach being a student as you would a job. Plan to be at it 40 hours a week. Small-business owners will tell you they average closer to 60 hours a week, and you qualify as a small business.

Don't make the mistake of thinking that because you have only one class on Tuesday and no class on Thursday, those are your "days off." Actually, those are the days when you can really get down to business. Although it is important to use every fragment of time, it is even more important to schedule large blocks of uninterrupted study time lasting 2 or 3 hours.

Concentration. One key to success is undivided attention. Eliminate all distractions. Clear your work area and your mind of all clutter. Keep on the desk only what you need for a particular assignment. If your mind wanders, order it back to the task at hand. Superstudents not only do first things first, they do only one thing at a time.

Dirty Jobs. Look at your to-do list and circle the task you dread doing most. Tackle that one first. When it is finished, you will feel exhilarated.

If you postpone doing a boring, tough, or unpleasant task, it will nag you all day. Your ability to concentrate will be nil. As the day wears on, you will begin to think about putting it off until tomorrow. That way the task will ruin two days instead of one. So take the plunge and do the dirty job first.

Equipment. Have a ready supply of pens, pencils, paper, note cards, computer disks, and printer ribbons or cartridges on hand. There is nothing more inconvenient than having to make a mad dash to an all-night convenience store.

Invest in the latest edition of each required textbook. Should you buy a used book? Buying a preowned book is like buying a used car. If the previous owner was a straight-A student, the yellow highlights and scribbles in the margins may be a godsend. Unfortunately, most straight-A students keep their books. The market is flooded with C-minus students' books. If your eye is easily distracted by another student's notes or highlighting, buy a new book.

To avoid frequent trips to the library for minor tidbits of information, build your own mini-reference library. Besides a standard dictionary and thesaurus, include a medical-nursing dictionary, drug handbook, *Merck Medical Manual*, and _____ (ask your instructors for suggestions to fill in the blank).

Filing System. With the "it-must-be-here-somewhere" filing system, you will not only lose time, you will lose your temper. Browse at the local bookstore for a filing system that meets your needs. If you can't afford what's in the store, go behind the store and get a sturdy cardboard box from the trash. Keep everything together. Put all papers pertaining to a certain class in one folder, and keep all folders for the current term in one box.

Once the term is over, take all those folders and move them to an under-the-bed storage box. That way the stuff will be out of sight but easily accessible. Then when your classroom studies are focused on the renal system, but you find yourself caring for a pregnant schizophrenic with a broken leg, you can quickly find your notes from last term or even last year.

Goals. Goals may be as simple as reading two chapters before bedtime or as complex as becoming a nurse-midwife in Borneo. Some take 10 minutes to accomplish; others take 10 years.

Being goal-oriented helps you focus your time and energy for maximum effect. It enables you to weed out irrelevant people and activities. Dozens of daily decisions become automatic.

If you find yourself wishing you could get a better grade in anatomy and physiology, or get into the clinical rotation at Children's Hospital next spring, or get more help with the housework, stop wishing and convert those wishes into goals. Sit down and work through the following:

1. List the steps you need to take to achieve the goal.
2. Decide which steps you are able to take to achieve the goal.
3. Decide which steps you are willing to take to achieve the goal.
4. Identify people who can help you achieve the goal.
5. Consider how you might let yourself or others sabotage your good intentions.

If you take the time to write down a goal and your plan for achieving it, you won't need a fairy godmother to make your dreams come true.

Hanging in There. When the going gets tough, hang in there. As the difficulty of any task increases, so does the attractiveness of any distraction. As you squirm in your chair, doing your laundry suddenly seems vital. Ignore the laundry. Knuckle down and work through the problem at hand. If you abandon a task when you feel you are losing, you'll find it much harder to return to it. Active avoidance coupled with passive procrastination will cost you lots of time. Instead, stop work at a point where you feel you are winning. Then you will be willing, even eager, to return to the task later.

Investments. Think of class attendance, library time, and study sessions as "deposits." Even brief moments, like small change, can add up to something big. One student tucked chemical formulas into her ski boot and memorized them on the chairlift.

Learn to Prioritize. Invest time in high-payoff activities. Required classes take priority over electives. Nursing classes take priority over any other class. Studying for an exam that makes up 50% of your grade takes precedence over studying for an exam that only makes up 10% of a grade. And so on.

Jotting it Down. Make lists and use them. It's the best way to stay organized and avoid wasted motion. Lists help you consolidate errands so that you make two trips instead of 20. Lists help you arrive prepared and ready for action.

Efficiency experts suggest you make a list each evening for the following day. List the six most critical things that have to be done. Rank them in order of importance. The next day, begin with number one and work it through before going on to anything else. Continue down the list. Your productivity will skyrocket.

Knocking Off. When you reach the point of diminishing returns, discontinue an activity. Settle for an A—don't knock your brains out striving for an A-plus. No one wastes more time than a perfectionist.

Remember Parkinson's law: "Work expands to fill the amount of time available to do it." Set reasonable deadlines and stick to them. Then move on to the next task.

Librarian. No one on campus can help you save as much time as the librarian. Just ask.

Majoring in Minor Activities. Busywork gives many students a false sense of accomplishment. Each night they fall into bed exhausted, insisting they are working as hard as they can. They're right. They're just not working as smart as they can.

Learn to recognize busywork for what it is. Don't take pride in your efforts. Take pride only in results.

"No". The greatest timesaving device ever invented.

Other People's Time. Time-wise students know how to divide chores and delegate everything they possibly can. They are also aware of some important considerations when relying on other people's time.

For example, if you are hiring someone to type your term paper, get the material to the typist well in advance of the due date. One campus typist, tired of last-minute hysterics, posted this notice on her wall: "A LACK OF PLANNING ON YOUR PART DOES NOT CONSTITUTE AN EMERGENCY ON MINE." If you are relying on other people's time, plan far ahead.

Prime Time. Every person has 2 or 3 hours a day when he or she is in top form. Most of us have our prime time in the morning.

Find your prime time and protect it. Invest it in high-priority items that demand concentration, creativity, and judgment. Use your less-than-prime time for legwork.

Questions. Several times each day, ask yourself questions such as the following:

- Is this the best use of my time right now?
- Is this activity helping me achieve one of my goals?
- Is this worth the amount of time it will take?
- Is this still worth doing?
- If I didn't do this, what would happen?

Regrets. Don't squander time mourning what might have been. Don't waste time wallowing in guilt or self-pity. When you begin to say, "If only," quickly change the statement to "Next time." Then get on with the business at hand.

Saving Time. Impossible! It is also impossible to find time or make time. You can only put the time you have to better use.

Tomorrow. It never comes. Do it TODAY.

Urgency! Urgent things are not always important. Important things are not always urgent. Tending to the important and ignoring the pseudoimportant things that clamor for attention are what separate good students from great students.

Vacillating. Indecision robs students of enough time to be classified as grand larceny. Be decisive. Establish your own operating policies. If you give yourself a deadline, stick to it. If you decide your regular study period will be from 2:00 to 4:00 PM, Monday through Friday, don't violate that policy. Studying anything is better than studying nothing.

Wastebasket. Use it!

Xeroxing. For dimes and quarters you can cut your library time to the bone. Use your less-than-prime time to round up all appropriate books and journals. Scan 2 minutes for articles, 3 minutes for books. Photocopy anything that appears pertinent. Use your prime time to study, memorize, integrate, synthesize, and use the information.

Keep copies of all your written papers and major assignments. If you prepared your assignment on a computer, be sure to save your work to the hard drive and a flash drive or CD. It's a dirt-cheap insurance policy against loss.

Yakety yak. Don't let the telephone or a drop-in visitor ruin your study time. Tell callers, "I can't talk right now. I'll call you back at 9 o'clock." If you can't do that, unplug the phone or go where there are no phones.

Close your door. If someone pops in and asks, "Have you got a minute?" say "No, but I'll have a minute at 9 o'clock." Offer to meet in his or her room or in the coffee shop. That way you can control the length of the visit.

Zzzzs. Schedule rest-and-relaxation periods. Get the sleep you need so you will be alert enough to put all these time management suggestions to good use.

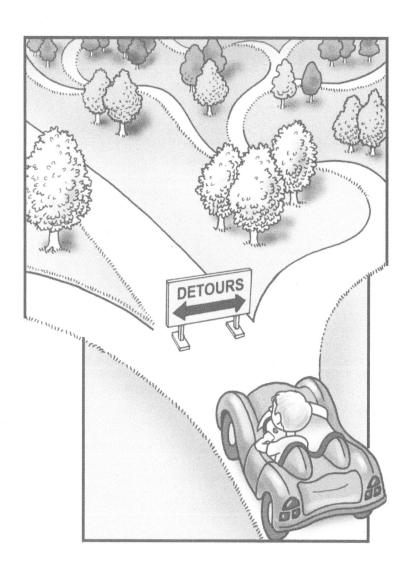

CHAPTER 11

Detours

"Time is the coin of life. It is the only coin you have, and only you can determine how it will be spent. Be careful lest you let other people spend it for you."
—CARL SANDBURG

Clutching your to-do list, you start off with the best intentions. Today you are really going to cover ground. There is a term paper to tackle, a chemistry quiz coming up, a patient to interview, some assigned journal articles to read, and a dental appointment at 3 o'clock. But first you'd better throw in a load of laundry (DETOUR). Then the phone rings (DETOUR).

Finally you are off and running. Rounding the first bend, you bump into an old friend who invites you for coffee (DETOUR). Now 2 hours behind schedule, you arrive at the library. Looking for the required journal articles, you happen upon a fascinating issue about career planning (DETOUR). That leaves time to read only three of the required articles before class.

After class you walk over to the hospital and find that your patient is unavailable. (He is always in physical therapy at this time of day.) Oh, well, you can kill some time in the cafeteria (DETOUR).

The patient interview takes longer than you expected, making you 15 minutes late for class. Embarrassed to walk in late, you decide to cut class (DETOUR). You go directly to chem lab and begin preparing for today's assignment.

Leaving lab a few minutes early, you dash to the dentist's office. You are on time, but he isn't. You are kept waiting for an hour. Unfortunately you left your chemistry notes at the lab, so you decide to write a long-overdue letter to your mom (DETOUR).

With half your face numb, you leave the dentist's office. You drive toward campus intending to start work on that term paper. Caught in rush-hour traffic, you suddenly feel drained. It has been a long day. You deserve an evening off. You turn around and head for home thinking, "There's always tomorrow" (DETOUR).

Know the Warning Signs

The word detour comes from the French meaning "to divert." Diversions come in all shapes, sizes, and disguises. Keeping on course requires constant attention. To avoid unnecessary detours, ask yourself several times a day: "Is what I am doing or about to do helping me reach one of my goals?" If the answer is no, you are on a detour.

Most students who fail to graduate aren't losers; they just get lost. They start out on the right road but forget where they are going. They lose sight of their goal. They are lured off the track by seemingly harmless diversions.

Always keep your eye on the finish line. Never forget that your NUMBER ONE GOAL IS TO GRADUATE.

Goals determine priorities. Priorities determine how you allocate such limited resources as time, money, and energy. Graduation is your long-term goal. All of your short-term goals should contribute directly or indirectly to that end.

The only way to graduate is to stay in school. The only way to stay in school is to successfully complete one test, one paper, one patient, one clinical skill, one term at a time. These are the minor goals that add up to your major goal.

Wishbones Versus Backbones

Students spend a lot of time wishing:

> "I wish my term paper were done."
> "I wish I could lose 10 pounds."
> "I wish I didn't procrastinate so much."
> "I wish I could get a better grade in chemistry."
> "I wish my family helped more with household chores."
> "I wish I could get into a different clinical group."

Converting a wish into a goal requires a workable plan. To formulate such a plan, ask yourself the five following questions:

1. What do I need to do to get what I want?
2. What am I willing to do to get what I want?
3. How will getting what I want affect my life?
4. Whom can I count on to help me get what I want?
5. How might I sabotage myself so I don't get what I want?

Let's take "I wish I could get a better grade in chemistry" and work it through from a wish to a goal.

1. What do I need to do to get a better grade in chemistry? I might need to do such things as:

   - Spend extra time studying chemistry assignments
   - Memorize formulas
   - Ask questions in class
   - Complete all assignments
   - Join a study group
   - Hire a tutor
   - Buy a study guide or supplementary textbook
   - Change lab partners
   - Ask the instructor for help
   - Do projects for extra credit

2. What am I willing to do to get a better grade in chemistry?

   Reading over the list I made in response to the first question, I circle those things I am willing and able to do to improve my grade. I will be scrupulously honest. There is no sense trying to kid myself.

   Knowing what has to be done and doing it are two different things. If I refuse to take the steps I have outlined, getting a better grade in chemistry remains a wish and never becomes a goal.

3. How will getting a better grade in chemistry affect my life?

   If I know what I have to do to get a better grade but am unwilling to take the necessary action, this question might give me the extra incentive I need. The results may be worth the effort if by improving my grade I can keep from flunking out, or raise my GPA, or increase my self-esteem and confidence.

   Because I cannot "find" time or "make" time, I am going to have to "take" time away from other activities. Shifting time to chemistry may mean getting up an hour earlier or going to bed an hour later. It may mean spending less time with friends and family. It may mean jeopardizing my grade in another course.

   My goals and priorities determine what I will do; they also determine what I will not do.

   This is the most difficult aspect of being a goal-oriented student. I am forced to admit that although I may be able to do anything, I simply cannot do everything. The ability to make tough decisions based on goals and priorities is what separates superstudents from so-so students.

4. Whom can I count on to help me improve my grade in chemistry?

   Me, myself, and I. That's three. Perhaps my instructor, a classmate, my spouse, the lab assistant, or a professional tutor. I will evaluate all possible human resources.

5. How might I sabotage myself so I don't get a better grade?

I might give up without even trying. I might continue to cross my fingers, close my eyes, and hope for the best. I might put off taking action until it is too late. I might rationalize by saying I cannot afford to put more time into chemistry, while not admitting that being unwilling to pay the price is not the same as being unable to pay the price of a higher grade.

By using these five questions, you can establish a plan for achieving any goal: completing a term paper, losing 10 pounds, improving grades, or getting more help around the house. Activating and sticking to the plan takes real backbone.

Goals to Go

Goals should be realistic and attainable. Don't become sidetracked by a compulsion for perfection. Some students want not only to graduate but also graduate with honors—or not at all. Settle for pure, unadulterated graduation. Don't take a difficult goal and make it impossible.

Goal-oriented students strive to make everything they do pay off in terms of long-range achievement. They may even take part-time jobs in the health care industry, thinking they will not only earn needed income but will also gain valuable experience.

Instructors advance strong arguments for and against such practice. The "pros" say such jobs provide flexible hours, give students a taste of the real world, boost confidence, and supplement the limited clinical experience provided by the school. The "cons" say such jobs are exhausting and usually pay poorly. The menial jobs offered to students provide meager clinical experience and imprint subordinate status, a mindset that is difficult to break.

Should you take a job in the health care industry while going through nursing school? Again, remember that your goal is to graduate. Choose the job that best contributes to that goal.

If you are thoroughly intimidated by the clinical setting, a hospital job may increase your confidence. As your confidence grows, your performance will improve. On the other hand, if you are floundering academically, stop working altogether or look for a low-stress job that allows time to study, such as being a desk clerk, night watchman, or dispatcher. When choosing your job, be practical. The better the salary, the fewer hours you have to work and the more time you can devote to your education.

Stick to business during business hours. Keep your eye focused on the finish line and you will take fewer detours. Keep evaluating each activity and assignment in terms of your goals. For example, is what you are doing at this very moment contributing to one of your goals? YES. Keep reading!

CHAPTER 12

You Can't Get There from Here

"A problem is nothing but concentrated opportunity."
—Dr. Norman Vincent Peale

After wandering through the New England countryside and becoming hopelessly lost, a motorist stopped and asked a farmer for directions. The farmer paused, then shook his head and replied, "You can't get there from here."

It's an old joke, but the punch line is one that nursing students hear all too often. When you find it necessary to ask for guidance and you are given a you-can't-get-there-from-here answer, don't believe it. Ask again. Ask someone else.

"I wanted to take a business course as an elective, but I didn't have the necessary prerequisite. My advisor suggested I choose something else. Instead, I went to the professor and told him what I hoped to gain from the class and why my life experiences should count as the prerequisite. He granted permission. It was one of the best classes I have ever taken."

Many students make the mistake of asking only one person—often not even the right person. Before you give up, get a second opinion and perhaps a third. Asking for what you want is no guarantee that you will get it, but not asking guarantees failure.

A nurse who wanted to work on her bachelor's degree had a list of lower-division courses she was required to take before she could proceed. To save money she thought she would take them at the community college instead of the university.

Luckily, her new faculty advisor was a former dean of students. When he interviewed her, he thought attending community college would be a waste of time and money. He encouraged her to make a list of her professional accomplishments, life experiences, and the training sessions she had attended. "Deans read better than they listen," he told her.

She returned to the university with her list in hand. She was immediately placed in upper-division courses. Not only did she save thousands of dollars, she saved a year and a half of her life!

If you are going to find your way from one end of nursing to the other, make sure you pack plenty of persistence. If one approach doesn't work, switch to another. Be bold enough to deal directly with the people involved and bright enough to bring concrete evidence.

"One of our instructors talked so fast we could not keep up with her. Several of us asked her to slow down, but within a few minutes she would be spewing forth facts and figures at an incomprehensible rate. Our test scores went down. Finally, we decided to record one of her lectures. We made an appointment and played the tape back to her. After listening she apologized and changed her style. Our test scores improved."

Instructors are not mind readers. If you need help, speak up.

"In one of our courses, 10 different teachers presented material. There was some conflicting information, and as the final exam drew closer, we got very worried. Whom could we trust for the correct answer? We asked all the teachers to attend a review session. We asked questions and finally got straight answers."

Faculty members are not purposely insensitive; they are just insanely busy. A major problem for you may look minor on their overcrowded to-do list. Instead of hoping the instructor will deal with your problem quickly, set a definite time. If you say, "I'll check back with you at 4 o'clock tomorrow," you will be less likely to get lost in the shuffle. When you show up the next day, you will either get your answer or reinforce the urgency of your need. It's better to find out that your problem has been overlooked for 24 hours than for 2 weeks. You may also try sending your instructor an e-mail or leaving a phone message or note.

When meeting a problem head on, a good way to rally support is to draft a petition. Follow proper channels and stick to your guns.

"Our library wasn't open on Sundays. We wrote a petition and virtually everyone signed it. The class officers presented it to the dean. We were given all sorts of excuses why it couldn't be done. We just kept pushing for it. Like when we were told the budget wouldn't allow it—all sorts of students volunteered to help staff on a rotating basis. Finally, they agreed to open for 4 hours on Sunday afternoons. Traffic in the library has been so heavy they are talking about expanding weekend hours next fall."

Complaining is always easier than generating creative alternatives. Before you call attention to a problem, have several possible solutions in mind. In the following situation the students didn't just let off steam, they proposed a way to streamline the system:

"We were required to write out six full nursing-care plans on our patients. Students were staying up so late and coming to clinical so tired they could not function very well. We asked the instructors if we could do some of our care plans orally. We figured you have to know your stuff thoroughly either way. The instructors agreed to a trial period. The new system worked so well that students and instructors voted to keep it going."

In all five of the above examples the students managed to "get there from here." You can be successful, too—IF you have the right kind of drive.

Psychology Behind the Wheel

By now you have noticed that students have very different driving styles. Some are passive. Some are aggressive.

You can always tell passive drivers by the tread marks on their backs. They are quiet, overly cautious, excessively polite, and indecisive. Always waiting to be told what to do and where to go, they create bottlenecks and are a menace to other drivers as well as to themselves.

Aggressive drivers are fast and reckless. They honk once, and if you don't get out of their way, they run right over you. Their hit-and-run techniques leave the nursing course looking like a demolition derby. They don't care who gets hurt as long as they get where they want to go.

Both passive and aggressive students have low self-esteem. Some have none.

As a student you occupy a subordinate role, and most of us have found that "subordinate" is a euphemism for "inferior." Even though you are not inferior, when you occupy the subordinate position, as in parent-child, employer-employee, doctor-nurse, teacher-student, you may begin to have self-doubts. You may feel inferior and behave in inferior ways.

For whatever comfort it is, this problem occurs at all levels of education. Students working on their master's degrees and doctorates experience similar feelings. They begin to question their intelligence and worth. It is just inherent in the role of student.

You don't have to be either passive or aggressive. You can choose a style that is neither reticent nor reckless. You can choose to be assertive.

The Assertive Lane

Assertiveness is an attitude, coupled with action, that allows you to move through traffic without being injured or injuring others. One way to become more assertive is to adjust your attitude. As your attitude changes, so will your actions.

To offset feelings of inferiority, try viewing your instructors as your employees. After all, you are paying them to teach you the fine art of nursing. They work for you. And, as an employer, you have the right to make requests; ask for improvements; evaluate work performance; and expect loyalty, courtesy, and prompt attention.

An easier way to become more assertive is to adjust your actions. As your behavior changes, so will your attitudes.

How do assertive students act? They stand tall, look you in the eye, and speak up. They are honest enough to express their feelings but tactful enough to protect your dignity. They will laugh with you but never at you. And they love to laugh at themselves.

They are not afraid to say:

"I prefer…"
"I dislike…"
"I am concerned…"
"I need…"
"I want…"
"I do not understand…
"I disagree…"
"I expect…"

Assertive students are able to accept compliments graciously. They are able to accept criticism thoughtfully. When they fail, they look on failure as a learning experience. Then they adjust their course and head off in a new direction.

When faced with tough problems, they look for solutions instead of scapegoats. They are not interested in plotting to get even because they are too busy planning to get ahead. They are not afraid to make decisions and actively pursue their goals.

Basically, assertive students are realists with optimistic overtones. They share common qualities: positive persistence, boldness, and confidence.

Many nursing schools have integrated assertiveness training into the curriculum. On the surface these skills appear so simple that many overlook the potential power of such a tool. Few appreciate the length of time it takes to become proficient with assertiveness: a lifetime.

Passive and aggressive students may survive the nursing curriculum, but only assertive students have the drive to thrive. The same is true of graduate nurses. Only assertive professionals thrive and consistently manage to "get there from here."

CHAPTER **13**

Drive-Up Teller

"Old Time, in whose banks we deposit our notes
Is a miser who always wants guineas for groats;
He keeps all his customers still in arrears
By lending them minutes and charging them years."
—OLIVER WENDELL HOLMES

If you are always in a hurry, you probably like the drive-up window at the bank. You can make transactions without leaving your car. But you still need to fill out the proper forms. You can't just throw money at the drive-up teller and expect it to land in your account.

The same is true of the Memory Bank. You can't just throw information in its general direction and expect to find it later in your account.

The Memory Bank has two branches: short-term and long-term. Cramming is like making a massive deposit in the short-term branch. As long as you withdraw it almost immediately, the lump sum remains intact. If you check on your account a week later, you will find that your deposit has dwindled. A month later you will find a considerable loss. Six months later the account will be closed.

If you want sufficient "funds" available when you go to write state board exams, you cannot rely on your short-term memory bank. The only way to stay solvent is to make deposits in the long-term branch.

The drive-up teller at the long-term branch is best at handling small, regular deposits. Every time you review information, you add to your account. When you review your account, you add interest.

If you tell yourself and others that you have a poor memory, you give your mind permission to forget. Another self-fulfilling prophecy comes true. Instead, tell yourself you have a good or even a great memory. Desire plus confidence pays big dividends.

Some things you think you've forgotten you never actually knew in the first place, such as when you don't quite catch a person's name but you nod and move on.

In the classroom you can't afford to nod and move on. If you don't quite catch the information, ask the instructor to spell the name of the drug or disease. If your notes say there are six common side effects but you can only account for five, ask for the sixth. Get complete, correct information and fix it firmly in your mind.

You cannot remember what you do not understand. One way to check your understanding is to paraphrase the information or think of examples to see whether you really grasp the principles involved.

Information must be meaningful if it is to be remembered. Merging the information with previous or present experiences enables it to be properly catalogued, stored, and retrieved for future use.

When classroom and clinical experiences are synchronized, memory is enhanced. Unfortunately the two are often out of synch. Merely reading about Huntington's chorea simply does not have the same effect as reading about it while caring for a patient with the disease.

Memorycise

Experts often compare memory to a muscle that improves with exercise. Stay in shape; work your memory. Experiment with various techniques such as visualization and mnemonics.

An example of visualization is picturing yourself paddling a microscopic canoe along the bloodstream. Envision passing through each chamber of the heart and navigating the entire system, down to the smallest capillaries. The more vivid or ludicrous the imagery, the more likely you are to remember.

Mnemonics is another key to opening the memory bank. For example, taking the first letter of each word in a series and forming a new word or phrase or a name such as Roy G. Biv may help you remember the order of the colors in the rainbow: red, orange, yellow, green, blue, indigo, and violet. Another way to remember a list of items is to make a sentence using the first letter of every word. Two common ones in the health sciences are (1) "On old Olympus' towering top, a Finn and German viewed a hop" and (2) "Never lower tiny perambulator, mamma might come home." The first sentence helps you remember the 12 cranial nerves (olfactory, optic, oculomotor, trochlear, trigeminal, abducens, facial, acoustic, glossopharyngeal, vagus, accessory, hypoglossal), and the second represents the bones of the wrist (navicular, lunate, triangular, pisiform, multangular/greater, multangular/lesser, capitate, and hamate).

If you want to amass a wealth of information, following are two ways to make deposits in the Memory Bank.

1. LISTENING AND LEARNING

To get the most out of the hours you spend in the classroom, follow these five rules: (1) show up, (2) sit in the front, (3) participate in class discussions, (4) ask questions, and (5) look alive! Arrive on time with all necessary equipment. Come rested, nourished, and eager. Choose a seat near the front, away from distractions. Lean forward. Smile. Make eye contact with the instructor. Concentrate. The more you can absorb during class time, the less you will have to absorb on your own time.

Because you are able to hear three times faster than most instructors are able to speak, your mind will have time to wander. Instead of doodling or daydreaming, use that time to organize your notes, differentiate between facts and opinions, fill in gaps, underline material emphasized, and think of practical applications.

During class listen to your inner voice. Are you criticizing the lecturer's ability or appearance? Are you busily refuting or belittling what is being said? When you study under a less-than-ideal instructor, you must make a conscious effort to separate the content from the person presenting it. Avoid running internal arguments or making snide comments to yourself. Listen and learn despite what you think of the instructor.

TAKE NOTES, but don't try to write down every word the instructor says. Few authors and even fewer lecturers are worth quoting verbatim. Before you move your pen, listen. Condense what is said and convert it into your own words. Five minutes of lecture may yield only five words.

Write legibly. Create your own shorthand, but be consistent so that you will be able to decipher it. Here are some abbreviations and symbols that can speed up your note taking and thus give you more time for listening.

♀	female
♂	male
>	greater than
<	less than
=	equals, the same
≠	does not equal, different
×	times
→	leads to, going
←	from, away
↑	up, increasing, above
↓	down, decreasing, under
$	dollar
$\bar{c}$	with
$\bar{s}$	without
⊕	positive
⊖	negative
Q.	question
A.	answer
q.	every
∴	therefore
∵	because
~	approximately
Hx	history
Dx	diagnosis
Rx	treatment, prescription

Use this space to write or draw other abbreviations and symbols you frequently use. Compare with classmates.

Make your notes fun to read. Use different colors of paper or ink. Toss in an occasional joke or cartoon.

Some students divide their notebook so that the left-hand page contains text notes and the right-hand page contains class notes. Others prefer separate notebooks for readings and lectures. In either case, leave generous margins where you can make study lists or insert new material.

After class, review your notes as soon as possible—take notes on your notes. Use the margins to summarize. Look for broad principles, see if you understand relationships, separate major from minor facts, assemble any lists worth memorizing, check for discrepancies between lecture and text, and write down questions that occur to you.

2. READING AND REMEMBERING

While reading a journal for nurse educators, an article title caught my eye: "The Relative Influence of Identified Components of Text Anxiety in Baccalaureate Nursing Students." TEXT anxiety? It was a typographical error missed by some proofreader asleep at the switch. The article was on test anxiety, not text anxiety.

But I quickly latched on to the idea. If there isn't a disorder called text anxiety, there should be. For example, adult health nursing textbooks average 2000 pages. They will soon have to come equipped with wheels because they're too heavy to carry around. Five years ago, a dozen consultants would be involved in producing a nursing text. Today as many as five dozen experts contribute to each textbook.

If your nursing books appear to be written in a foreign language, they are. They are written in Latin mixed with technical jargon. Instead of skipping over unfamiliar words, flip to the glossary at the back of the text and keep a medical-nursing dictionary close at hand.

Immerse yourself in the language. Study common root words, suffixes, and prefixes. Make flash cards and carry them with you (see Appendix A).

As you struggle to learn this new language, be acutely aware of your feelings and frustrations. Once you begin speaking "medicalese" like a native, it is easy to forget what patients and their families go through as they struggle to understand us.

As a nursing student you will have not only a horrendous amount of reading but also a horrendous amount of hard reading. Educators use a formula based on the length of words and sentences to assess the relative difficulty of written material and assign a grade level to it. For example, *Reader's Digest* requires grade 8 reading ability, and the *Wall Street Journal* requires grade 10 ability. Nursing students in one baccalaureate program used the formula on their medical-surgical text and found that it required grade 17 ability! When you need 5 years of college to understand a required freshman text, you realize the importance of reading skills.

If you are a poor reader, you will need help sharpening your skills or else you will not survive the nursing curriculum. Ask about programs to improve reading speed and comprehension. Commercial courses are available, but they are usually expensive. Your school may offer a comparable course for much less and may even give you college credit for it.

Here are some tips to help you get more out of your reading time:

Before You Begin Reading

Pick a place with no distractions, or if you're in your room, padlock the refrigerator, turn off the TV, disconnect the phone, and hang a DO NOT DISTURB sign on the door. Sit at a desk so you can take notes. Choose a chair that is comfortable but not too comfortable. You don't want to doze off. If you need glasses, wear them, and always make sure you have sufficient light.

Ask yourself why you are reading this particular material. Consult the chapter objectives if they're provided. Decide whether your mission is to uncover facts, understand principles, answer specific questions, assess relevance, or create a term paper or a research project of your own.

Before reading the first paragraph, take a couple of moments to skim the entire chapter or article. To understand what the author considers important, look at section headings, any bold type, italicized words, illustrations, diagrams, charts, or graphs. Read the whole summary. Examine the study questions provided. To understand what your instructor considers important, check the course outline, objectives, study questions, and any handouts pertaining to this assignment.

While You Read

Don't just go through the motions. Remember that it's not what you put into reading, it's what you get out of it that counts. The best way to remember what you read is to take notes. A much less effective way is to use a highlighter or to underline as you read. Reading by itself is a poor third choice.

Instruct your mind to focus on the material. Watch for connecting words, qualifiers, and punctuation marks that can completely change the meaning. Reread difficult passages slowly. Move your lips. Reading aloud can increase comprehension.

Read to understand, not to memorize. As you take notes, put the material in your own words. If you can put the material in your own words, you understand it. If you understand it, you can remember it.

Vary your speed. (Average reading speed varies from 100 to 400 words per minute.) One of the quickest ways to improve speed and comprehension is to use your fingertips to "underline" the sentences as you read. A comfortable position is to turn your palm up and use your middle and index fingers. This action pulls your eyes along the page, enabling you to see more words at a time. It also reduces the chances of losing your place or staring at one word while your mind goes elsewhere.

Maintain a positive attitude. Try to keep an open mind. Resist the urge to argue with the author. If you find statements that seem contradictory or confusing, place a question mark in the margin and ask the instructor for clarification.

After Reading

Quickly review your notes or scan what you have underlined in the text. Try to sum up the chapter in your own words. Take a second look at any illustrations, charts, or diagrams. Can you explain them without rereading? Can you answer the author's study questions? Your instructor's study questions?

Parking all this information in your long-term memory requires a chemical change to take place in your brain. Excessive physical or emotional activity immediately after a study session can interfere with this process. Instead of going to a football game or fighting with your spouse, put your book under your pillow and sleep on it.

When you check your statement from the long-term memory bank, you will find that you remember every "first" with remarkable clarity—your first patient, your first injection, your first day in surgery. You are also likely to find any information that startled, surprised, amused, or interested you. And you will have total recall of everything your instructor prefaced with, "You don't have to know this for the test but...." Bank on it!

CHAPTER 14

Tollbooth

"By failing to prepare, you are preparing to fail."
—Benjamin Franklin

Zooming along, you spot a tollbooth. The tollgate is down; the red light is flashing. To go from Aspiring Nurse 101 to Aspiring Nurse 202, you have to come up with the correct change: adequate scores on examinations, finished term papers, evidence of clinical competence, and a suitable GPA.

If you search your pockets and come up short, you may be able to persuade the gatekeeper to let you postpone payment. With an INCOMPLETE in hand you are allowed to "pass."

Don't delude yourself into thinking you can easily make up for lost time on the next leg of the course. Each leg is more difficult than the last, and if you are already pushing hard just to keep up, there will be almost no time for making up.

If you are not seriously ill and no one in the family is dying, it is far better to buckle down and complete this term now. Cut out the frills, get a tutor, burn the midnight oil, forget perfection, and accept a grade that is a notch lower than you'd like. Don't try to carry this term's work into next term.

Testing takes a heavy toll on many students. As test time approaches, they experience headaches, dizziness, diarrhea, insomnia, nausea, and assorted muscle cramps. No amount of studying reduces the panic. During the first few moments of the exam, they literally lose their minds. Everything goes blank.

"I was a babbling nervous wreck, flapping around the room like a wild animal, pouring sweat and unable to concentrate on any one thought for more than two or three seconds at a time."
—Hunter S. Thompson, *Fear and Loathing in Las Vegas*

Everyone experiences some degree of test anxiety. What may surprise low-performance students is that high-performance students experience the very same physical symptoms, but they instruct their minds not to pay any attention to them. Instead they focus on the test. They quickly become absorbed in the task at hand, and their physical symptoms disappear. High-performance students don't worry about how they are doing; they concentrate on what they are doing.

If you begin to panic during an exam, close your eyes for a moment. Breathe slowly and deeply. Talk positively to yourself. Knock off the easy questions first. This builds confidence and helps you perform to the best of your ability on the remainder of the test.

If you know a student who suffers from such extreme test anxiety that it would be more properly called "test terror," get him or her professional help.

High-performance students automatically use some simple skills that boost their scores. If you are a student who knows the material as well as your study partners, yet you consistently score lower than they do, these skills can help you even the score.

Preparation for Testing

High-performance students find out everything they can about the teacher and the test. First, they study the teacher. Is this instructor bent on helping students succeed or on weeding out as many students as possible? Is this a person obsessed with trivia or one who concentrates on principles, ideas, and relationships? What are this person's special interests and areas of expertise?

Second, they gather all the information they can about the test. What kind of test will it be? Multiple choice or essay? What material will be covered? Text and lecture only, or other reading assignments and laboratory work as well?

The best source of information on the test is the teacher. Just ask! Most are perfectly willing to share this information. You may also find it helpful to ask former students.

An excellent way to prepare for a new test is to study an old one. You may be surprised to learn that many instructors leave copies of their old tests on file at the library or in the department office. Even if the instructor has changed, chances are the course content hasn't. Many questions will be reworded but recognizable.

Believe it or not, you are better off with a teacher who gives frequent tests and quizzes. If there are only two tests given all term, too much is riding on each. By the time you figure out the teacher's style, it is almost too late to improve your grade. If you have a teacher who skimps on tests, it becomes even more important to track down everything possible about the exam beforehand.

When is the best time to begin studying for exams? The first day of class. Successful students attend class religiously, listen intently, take careful notes, and mark information the instructor emphasizes for special study. Soon after each class they condense their notes and review them frequently. (For more study tips see Chapter 10, "More Miles Per Gallon.")

Begin studying for a specific test 2 or 3 weeks in advance. Remember these words: READ * WRITE * REVIEW * RECITE. As you read, write! Don't just underline. Jot down the main facts, names, dates, ideas, and relationships. Put everything in your own words. If you can do that, you understand it. If you understand it, you can remember it. Review what you've written. Condense your notes. Reread them as often as possible. Close your text or notebook and recite what you have learned.

Most students find it helpful to study for tests with a partner or a small group. You often discover things you may have overlooked or underemphasized. When you coach other students, you get a better grasp of the material yourself.

Some major tests are not given in the regular classroom. Find out where the test will be given. Visit the room and actually spend time studying there. The more comfortable you are in the test room, the more relaxed you will be and the better you will perform.

24 HOURS BEFORE THE TEST

Keep food intake and exercise on the light side. Lay out equipment you want to take with you: pens, pencils, erasers, scratch paper, blue books, calculator, wristwatch, sweater, and—if it is a long test—a snack such as candy, peanuts, or raisins.

Surround yourself with pleasant, positive people. Avoid situations that depress or aggravate you.

10 MINUTES BEFORE THE TEST

Arrive at the test site 10 minutes before the exam. That's enough time to relax and not enough time to panic. Choose a seat away from windows, doors, aisles, friends, and enemies. If you are left-handed, make sure you get a left-handed desk.

Breathe slowly and deeply. Tense and relax your muscles, especially those in your neck and shoulders. Give yourself a pep talk, not an ultimatum.

DURING THE TEST

Listen carefully to oral instructions. Ask for clarification if you are confused. Read written instructions carefully. Take time to work through any sample questions provided. It will save you time in the long run.

Skim the entire test. How many questions are there? How much time can you allow for each? Are the questions weighted differently? For example, 100 multiple-choice questions may be worth only 40% of the grade, the matching section worth 10%, and the two essay questions worth 50%. Divide your time accordingly.

If marking on the test is allowed, scribble things you are afraid you will forget—names, dates, formulas, principles—on one of the corners. Circle or underline key words and phrases in the instructions. Examine the stem of each question for significant phrases such as "same as," "opposite of," or "only one."

Work quickly. Leave the toughies and time wasters for last. Remember that many answers are found or alluded to in other questions. Keep your eyes open.

A word of caution: Because you will be skipping over some questions, periodically check to make sure the number on the question and the number on the answer sheet match.

TIPS FOR MULTIPLE-CHOICE ITEMS

- Read directions carefully.
- Work quickly. Put a star or checkmark by questions you want to return to later if you have time.
- Formulate your own answer before you read the answers given.
- Read every given answer.
- Eliminate implausible answers.
- Watch for absolutes and qualifiers. Answers containing "always," "never," "all," or "none" are usually incorrect.
- In many nursing exams multiple-choice questions are related to rather lengthy case studies. To avoid delays caused by rereading, scan all questions before reading the case study. Then your eyes will be more attuned to the important information.

TIPS FOR TRUE-FALSE ITEMS

- The longer the true-false statement, the more likely it is to be TRUE.
- There are usually more TRUE statements because they are easier to write.
- Most statements come verbatim from text or lecture. If it looks familiar, play your hunch.
- Statements containing "all," "only," "always," or "because" are usually FALSE.
- Statements containing "none," "generally," or "usually" are more often TRUE.

- If the statement is long or complicated, break it into smaller parts. Remember that if one part is false, the whole statement is FALSE.
- Don't change answers. On true-false items your first impression is usually correct.

TIPS FOR MATCHING ITEMS

- Check to see whether answers are used only once or more than once.
- Do easy matches first.
- Work down the column with the longest phrases.
- Look for patterns: dates-events, terms-definitions, people-contributions.

TIPS FOR SHORT ANSWER AND FILL-IN-THE-BLANK ITEMS

- Look for clues in language and sentence construction.
- The length of the blank usually indicates the length of the answer desired.
- If you know two possible answers, give both. You will rarely be penalized, and you may get extra credit.
- Make an educated guess. Don't leave the blankety-blank blank.

TIPS FOR MATHEMATICAL ITEMS

- Read each question very carefully. Write down the givens, what you are expected to find, and any formulas you plan to use.
- Estimate the answer before doing calculations so you'll know whether you're close or far afield.
- Write legibly, and keep numbers in distinct columns.
- Copy accurately.
- Check units of measure—ounces, drams, millimeters.
- Use a calculator and any other aids and devices permitted.
- If abstractions confuse you, substitute simple numbers for symbols.
- Check math by working the problem backward.
- If the answer is in multiple-choice form and you haven't the foggiest idea, you can usually eliminate the highest and lowest answers given.

TIPS FOR ESSAY ITEMS

- When you are offered a choice of essay questions, read all of them before deciding which to tackle.
- Beside each question, quickly list the facts and ideas that pop into your head.

- Budget your time. Spend 50% outlining the answer and 50% writing it.
- Know who will be grading the exam. If it will be scored by a teaching assistant, forgo fancy writing and stuff every name, date, fact, idea, and key phrase you can remember into the answer.
- Underline key words in directions. Know precisely what you are to do. For example:

Summarize
Means to give a concise review of the main ideas.
Explain
Means to give the how or why of something.
Illustrate
Means to give effective examples.
Discuss
Means to explain and elaborate.
Define
Means to explain the meaning.
List
Means to give a series of items or ideas without elaborating.
Outline
Means to write only main ideas or facts.
Compare
Means to show similarities.
Contrast
Means to show differences.

- Organize your essay: title, topic sentence, main body, and conclusion.
- Make a final check for mechanics and spelling if time permits.
- If you run out of time, write "I ran out of time. Please accept my outline." You will get partial credit, and you may even get full credit.

QUESTIONABLE ITEMS

- If you are totally confused, don't panic. Ask the test monitor for clarification.
- Don't let toughies derail you. Move on to the next question. Your unconscious mind will go to work on the tough one while your conscious mind works on the next one. Something in another question may jog your memory or clear up confusion.
- Break long, complicated questions into small, manageable parts. Read slowly, moving your lips or subvocalizing each word.
- If two answers seem correct, choose the more obvious.
- If no answer looks correct, choose the most nearly correct answer.
- Give the answer the instructor wants. Don't quibble!

- Always guess unless there is a penalty for guessing (i.e., more points are subtracted for giving a wrong answer than for giving no answer), in which case, play the odds.
- If you wish to protest an item, see the instructor after the test but before grades are given out.

JUST BEFORE TURNING IN YOUR TEST

- Erase all stray marks on the answer sheet.
- Make sure that your name is on each sheet.
- Reread directions.
- Look at any questions you have flagged for further consideration. If you honestly believe an answer should be changed, change it. You will probably be correct. Just don't waffle back and forth and back again.
- Fill in all the blanks.
- Use all the time available.
- Never give up.

Final Tollbooth: National Council Licensure Exam (NCLEX®)

Taking some college courses is like being vaccinated. Once you've given it a shot and passed, you are "immune." Even if you can't remember anything from the course 2 weeks after the final, you never have to take the course again. For courses like that you can cram. In 3 days you can learn everything you need to pass the course, and 3 days later you can forget it all.

Nursing isn't like that. You will not only be required to remember, you will be required to understand virtually everything from your basic nursing courses. You will be expected to build on that information in more advanced courses, and every day you will apply what you've learned as you care for patients. The study of nursing demands continual review. There is no way to cram and survive.

Even after you have successfully completed all your schooling, there is still one final exam standing between you and your license to practice nursing. It is called NCLEX®-RN or "state boards." You'll learn more about it in Chapter 29. It will be unlike any other test. For now, all I can say is the best time to begin studying for the final to end all finals is the first day—and every day—of class.

CHAPTER 15

Totaled

"It's not the load that breaks you down, it's the way you carry it."
—LENA HORNE

"I failed! Now I'll never be a nurse!"

Hold on. Before you declare yourself a total wreck, take a closer look at the damage. You may not require a tow truck. You may just need some emergency road service.

If you've flunked an exam, bombed on a term paper, been chewed out by an instructor, or had an irate patient demand to see a "real" nurse, it can be devastating, but it is far from fatal.

Most failures signal a need for change, not an end to all your career aspirations. A poor performance in the classroom or clinical area warns you that things are not going as they should. Heed the warning.

The first step is to determine exactly what happened. Is this an isolated incident or a symptom of an underlying problem? Occasionally, failure is due to circumstances beyond your control. Occasionally.

To fail has several different meanings. For example, to fail means:

- To lose strength; to fade away or die away; to stop functioning
- To fall short
- To become absent or inadequate; to be deficient
- To disappoint the expectations or trust of someone

Let's look at how each of these meanings applies to the most common reasons for student failure, and explore possible remedies.

"To Lose Strength, to Fade Away or Die Away, to Stop Functioning"

LACK OF COMMITMENT

Lack of commitment is the number one reason for failure. Becoming a nurse is not a driving passion. Either you have temporarily lost sight of your goal or you have changed goals—consciously or unconsciously. Your interest is waning. You don't really hate nursing, but you don't really love it. You are lukewarm, and it is beginning to show in your grades.

Remedy: Everyone has a slump now and then. You may need a good night's sleep, a vitamin supplement, a day by the seashore, or a pep talk from a nurse who loves her work. For lingering slumps, talk with your advisor or a guidance counselor. It may be wise to voluntarily step out of school for a while rather than have failure make your exit mandatory.

LAZINESS

Becoming a nurse is requiring a lot more work than you ever imagined. Frankly you can't summon up the vim, vigor, and vitality required to keep pace with the rest of the class.

Remedy: Shove it in gear or start looking for a less demanding way to make a living.

ILLNESS

Sudden illness in yourself or a family member can throw a monkey wrench in the best-laid plans. Student nurses are on such an "unforgiving" time schedule that a few days out of commission can spell disaster.

Remedy: If the interruption is brief and you can get up to speed quickly, you may be able to catch up and finish the term successfully. If not, negotiate with the individual instructors for an "Incomplete" or an alternate assignment. Talk with your advisor about all the options. Check on the school's policy regarding withdrawal without penalty. Before you take the off-ramp, make sure there is an on-ramp available. Once off the track, you may be out of the course for a year or more.

"To Fall Short"

LACK OF ABILITY

Caring about sick people is one thing; caring for them is quite another. Nursing demands peak performance physically, mentally, and emotionally. You may be intellectually gifted but a basket case emotionally. You may be emotionally strong but physically frail. Not everyone has the right mix of talents, skills, and abilities to make a success of nursing.

Remedy: Determine which limitation is causing the failure. You can shore up sagging abilities, but it may require an inordinate amount of time and energy. Decide whether you are willing and able to take the corrective action. Seek professional counsel.

SELF-DEFEATING BEHAVIORS

Self-defeating behaviors might be more accurately called "imagined lack of ability." If you expect to fail, you will rarely be disappointed. Pessimists, nit-pickers, worrywarts, perfectionists, and procrastinators are some who fit into this category.

Remedy: Sometimes just recognizing a self-defeating behavior can change its impact so dramatically that you can convert failure into success. Other times these behaviors are so entrenched that professional help is required to overcome their crippling effects.

"To Become Absent or Inadequate; to be Deficient"

ABSENTEEISM

When Woody Allen was asked the secret of his success, he quipped that showing up was 80%. Students who fail are those who fail to show up for class. Grades are directly correlated with class attendance.

Remedy: Force yourself to attend every class. Sit near the front.

POOR STUDY HABITS

College students have to run full speed just to keep up. If your study skills are not up to snuff, your workload will be doubled. Not only will you have to master the subject matter, you will have to master study skills as well. By the time you realize the importance of being efficient and effective in your study habits, it may be too late. The damage will be done.

Remedy: Habit is the key word. Habitual study. Consistently putting in time with the books is vital if you are to survive. Knowing how to get the most out of your study time will help you thrive. For extra help, see Chapters 10, 13, and 14.

OUTSIDE ACTIVITIES

Although outside activities can greatly enrich your life, an overdose can kill you. The famous last words of many former students who failed to graduate are, "Never let school interfere with your education."

You may be a first-time-away-from-home student who is intoxicated by your new freedom. You are so busy experiencing life that you haven't had time to think about grades. Or you may be a superstudent, who edits the school paper, serves as council president, builds the homecoming float, and works 20 hours a week as a clerk. Or you may be the midlife mother-wife, promising that nothing will change just because you've added being a student to your already busy schedule. You still manage to keep the house spotless, teach Sunday school, manage the charity bazaar, and turn out gourmet meals when entertaining.

The only thing wrong with outside activities is that they gobble up time, and time is an irreplaceable resource. An A in homecoming, parenting, or partying will not balance an F in anatomy, microbiology, or organic chemistry.

Remedy: Recognize that to succeed as a student you will have to limit outside activities for a few years. Reevaluate the people, events, and things in your life. Simplify, simplify, simplify. Stick with a couple of the most satisfying activities, and slough off everything else.

"To Disappoint the Expectations or Trust of Someone"

Perhaps the most difficult aspect of failure is having to face all those people who expected you to become a nurse. Your parent or spouse says, "I don't understand. Why are you dropping out? You've wanted to be a nurse since you were 6 years old."

What do you say to people like that? First, remind them that you aren't 6 years old anymore, and suggest that no one should be bound by career choices made in childhood. "Yes, I always dreamed of being a nurse, but now I'm awake. And when I looked at nursing with my eyes wide open, I realized it wasn't the career for me."

Some things are more attractive from a distance, such as a beautiful suit that catches your eye from clear across the store. It looks great on the hanger, but when you try it on it just doesn't fit.

You've tried on nursing. It doesn't fit. Minor alterations are always possible, but major alterations may be impossible—or at the very least, impractical.

Remedy: Whether you failed nursing or nursing failed you, give yourself time to grieve. Loss is always painful, even if it is only a dream that has died. Then get out and shop around for a career that does fit. Someday when you are a successful lawyer, architect, teacher, mechanic, musician, or florist, a nurse will walk by and you'll say with a sigh, "There but for the grace of God [and a few lousy grades] go I."

•••

A nursing professor is serving on a board of directors with a former student to whom she gave a failing grade in a leadership course years before. In retrospect, the professor attributes the failure to her own inexperience as a teacher at the time and the student's nonconformity, which was misinterpreted by the faculty.

Today that former student is not only a nurse but also heads a multimillion-dollar company. And she failed LEADERSHIP!

Neither has mentioned the incident, and frankly, it is driving the professor nuts. I suggested she take her former student to lunch and have a good laugh over it. That failure may have been the catalyst that drove the student to success. After all, the best revenge is living well.

CHAPTER **16**

How to Jump-Start Your Battery

"Effective executives have learned that what one postpones one abandons."
—Peter Drucker

Have you ever jumped into your car and found the battery dead as a doornail? If you were parked on a hill, you may have tried this simple trick: You let the car start rolling, popped the clutch, and the engine leaped to life.

Sometimes you jump into a term paper and find it dead as a doornail. You sit at the computer, fingers poised, but nothing happens. The words won't come.

Instead of sitting immobilized for lack of the right words, type any words: random thoughts, sentence fragments, even gibberish. Don't waste time agonizing over the opening paragraph; skip to the middle section. Begin anywhere you can. Get rolling, pop the clutch, and your engine will leap to life. Remember, it is easier to steer a moving vehicle, and it is easier to edit than to write.

Have you ever found yourself reading the same sentence for the third time? That's a sure sign your battery is dead. You need to recharge before you continue. Get up and splash some cool water on your face. Stretch. Reach for the ceiling, then bend over and touch your toes. Do a dozen jumping jacks. Then sit down and begin reading again.

Does this sound familiar? "I know I should work on my care plan, but I just don't feel like it right now." Forget feelings. MOVE! Put the machinery in motion, and the feeling will follow.

If you are sitting idle alongside the road, here is one way to jump-start your battery. Take your kitchen timer and set it for 5 minutes. Pick up that required reading, your research notes, or the care plan you have to do, and agree to work on it for just 5 minutes. You can stand anything for 5 minutes, right?

In that few moments something miraculous usually happens. The most inert students are energized. When the timer rings, odds are you will continue the activity. You won't even want to quit.

Another way to conquer procrastination is to make an appointment with yourself. Select a definite day, time, and place to begin working on a project. Keep that appointment.

The Psychology of Putting it Off

Almost every student procrastinates. Some do it because they are rebellious. They hate being told what to do and when to do it. By refusing to meet deadlines, they experience a temporary high and a fleeting feeling of being in charge.

Others are thrill seekers. They see the deadline as the edge of a cliff. Driving pell-mell, they see how close they can come to the edge before chickening out. At the last minute they veer off and hurriedly do the project.

Some students love to experiment. They want to see whether the instructor really means DEADline or whether special privileges will be granted to keep them from a fatal plunge.

Still others use procrastination to protect their fragile egos. Endorsing the "I-work-better-under-pressure" theory, they try to cram 2 weeks of work into 2 days. In the last few hours they exert superhuman effort. If the project fares well, it affirms their better-under-pressure theory. If the project fares poorly, they comfort themselves with the thought that they could have done better. There just wasn't enough time. Afraid to really put their ability to the test, they continue to procrastinate. After all, wouldn't it be mortifying to work all term and produce only a mediocre project?

Out of Neutral and into Gear

If you are struggling to overcome procrastination, here is another gimmick to help you get moving. Take a piece of paper and fold it in half. On the right-hand side list everything you have to gain by completing a project on time or ahead of schedule. On the left-hand side list everything you have to gain by putting the project off until the last possible moment.

If you are honest, you will have to admit that the only things gained by procrastination are anxiety, guilt, low grades, and other assorted headaches. If you tackle projects promptly and aim for early completion, your grades will rise along with your self-confidence and self-esteem. You will experience relief, joy, a sense of accomplishment, and a certain amount of smugness. You will be able to take time off for good behavior and really enjoy yourself.

Time off is one thing procrastinators actually don't have. Undone work, unmet deadlines, and the dread of facing irate instructors haunt their leisure hours. Every time they pass the library or glance at their dusty keyboards, they suffer pangs of guilt. Constantly nagged by the thought of what they should be doing, they find it almost impossible to relax.

If you are a particularly stubborn procrastinator, you may have to use the carrot-and-stick approach. This method moves stubborn students as well as stubborn mules. For example, to get students moving, instructors dangle "carrots" in front of them, such as smiles, praise, recognition, good grades, merit scholarships, a spot on the dean's list, and opportunities for choice assignments. For "sticks" they use frowns, criticism, harassment, low grades, probation, and failure.

Some students respond more quickly to carrots; others, to sticks. How about you?

To get yourself moving, you can devise your own system of rewards and punishments. When you keep regular study hours or perform assignments promptly, reward yourself. Take a bubble bath, have lunch with a friend, watch your favorite TV program, have a cup of gourmet coffee, read the next chapter in a bestseller. If you fail to keep regular study hours or to meet a deadline, punish yourself. Take a cold shower, unplug the TV set, go without coffee, do a chore you despise, eat a bologna-banana sandwich.

To be most effective, your reward and punishment system must be highly individualized. One student's reward is another's punishment. Create your own list (see p. 96).

Just like this list, batteries have positive as well as negative poles. Whenever you need a jump-start, use one of your carrots, one of your sticks, or a combination of the two.

Check your battery frequently. If you begin to feel run-down, recharge by taking a different route home, eating supper at breakfast time, sending yourself roses, watching a vintage movie, wading in a brook, or diving into a new adventure.

Don't forget that batteries also run down when you turn off your engine but leave your lights on. Turn off your lights. Get some sleep.

CARROTS	STICKS
People, places, things, and activities I enjoy	People, places, things, and activities I dislike

CHAPTER **17**
10-4, Good Buddy

"All for one, one for all, that is our device."
—ALEXANDRE DUMAS, *The Three Musketeers*

Back in the dark ages, before there were cell phones, truckers used CB radios to talk to one another as they rambled over long stretches of road. Even though each trucker was alone, he or she was never lonely. There was great camaraderie.

Truckers kept each other apprised of road conditions, traffic accidents, speed traps, and places to find cheap gas and good eats. Conversation kept them awake. By forming convoys they could draft another truck and save fuel. When they signed off, they would say, "10-4, Good Buddy," meaning message received.

Long, lonely stretches of road loom between you and graduation. No one can possibly know the trials and tribulations you are going through. No one except *another nursing student.* That's why the best way to keep on truckin' is to form a convoy.

In a project sponsored by the University of San Francisco to help retain freshman nursing students, faculty members were surprised to learn how much homesickness was a factor in a student's decision to leave school. The first couple of months are the hardest. This is especially true for students who can't get home on weekends because of time, distance, or money problems. To curb the effect of homesickness, the project members suggested linking lonely students together, sponsoring group activities on weekends, or having a local student invite a stranded student home with him or her. Just letting the homesick students know that what they were feeling was normal and temporary helped a lot.

Some of their other suggestions to help freshman nursing students survive included having group and individual counseling sessions, having an intensive orientation program to help students sharpen their study skills and time management abilities, getting the new students involved with upperclassmen in the nursing school, encouraging participation in fun activities as well as study groups, and assisting them with personal problems as well as academic difficulties.

Marc Fisher, a columnist for the *Washington Post,* wrote about how the city government had planted 21 trees in his neighborhood and 6 months later all had died. In contrast, he told about a nearby neighborhood where 120 trees had been planted at the same time. All were alive and well. What made the difference?

One woman. Her name is Penny Moser. She attached a plastic pouch to each of the 120 trees with a note that said, "Hello, I'm your new tree. Please could you adopt me?" Inside the pouch was an information sheet that explained that to survive the first year, the tree needed to be watered at least once a week. Most of the trees were quickly adopted as people signed up to be the "foster parents." Even the "orphans" were watered regularly.

To survive the first year, students need to be watered and nourished. Some schools do a better job of that than others. At Catholic University in Washington, D.C., former dean Ann Marie Brooks enlisted alumni to adopt students. Each student was paired with a sponsor/mentor who was to follow him or her through the whole 4 years. Maybe she should have had them wear signs saying, "Hello, I'm your new nursing student. Please could you adopt me?"

If you are ever feeling lonely and overwhelmed, you might enjoy this wonderful Emily Dickinson poem titled "I'm Nobody! Who Are You?"

I'm Nobody! Who are you?
Are you—Nobody—Too?
Then there's a pair of us?
Don't tell! They'd advertise—you know!
How dreary—to be—Somebody!
How public—like a Frog—
To tell one's name—the livelong June—
To an admiring Bog!

Nursing students often band together to survive. Without the buddy system, many simply would not make it. When you have to drive in the dark as much as nursing students do, it's reassuring to hear a friendly voice and know you are not alone. Even though you know you must haul your own load, the trip is safer and more enjoyable when you share the road with others.

Safety in Numbers

Traveling with a group reassures you that you are on the right road. Just knowing you are not alone keeps panic at a manageable level. As you exchange ideas and experiences, your confidence grows.

The group helps you clear up mysteries, distinguish facts from rumors, set priorities, and achieve goals. Good buddies not only cheer you up when you are losing, they cheer you on when you are winning.

Belonging to a group has several other advantages:

- Working together facilitates problem solving.

"I am in a support group consisting of older students with children. We were all frantically trying to keep our stress levels down and our time-management skills up. After we formed the group, we found we could help each other solve problems on the home front as well as in the classroom. We encourage each other to take 1 day at a time, to prioritize, to do only what needs to be done, and not to hesitate to ask for help—at home or in school."

- Camaraderie replaces competition.

"Joining a study group was the best thing I ever did. I learned to compete with myself, not with other students."

- Group membership fosters cooperation.

"Instead of every student carrying a whole satchel of books to the clinical area, each student in our group carries a different one. That way all of our books are available for reference, but no one gets a broken back. Besides, there's not enough room in the clinical area to store any more of those 40-pound books!"

- Studying with a group means less chance of overlooking or missing important material.

"Our instructors all talk so fast that I knew I was missing things that were important. In study group I spend a few moments comparing my notes with classmates' notes. That way I can fill in the blank spots. My grades have really improved since I started studying with a group."

Strength in Numbers

If you're on your own, you may hesitate to challenge a school policy, call the instructor's attention to inconsistencies, or make special requests. Group support can give you courage.

"We were faced with so much material for each test that we were overwhelmed. We approached the instructors and told them we wanted to have four tests instead of two. And they went for it!"

- Studying with friends can lift not only your spirits, but also your GPA.

"I was disappointed in my grade in micro. I thought I had a B going for me, but I received a C. When I mentioned it in my study group, they insisted I talk with the instructor and report back. I did get a B! (There was a computer error.) Without group support and encouragement, I would never have approached the instructor."

- Groups can decrease depression and increase productivity.

"Our class was always bitching and complaining about the heavy workload, the tedious assignments, etc. Some of us decided to form a study group with one rule: No bitching. Instead of complaining about tiresome assignments, we figure out ways to do them better and faster than if we tried to do them alone. We make lists, cross out days on the calendar, and generally encourage each other to think positively. Things still aren't perfect, but we're a lot less depressed."

If you aren't already in a study group, shop around for one. If you can't find one, start one. If you're hesitant, just try it out and see how you like it. For example, organize a temporary group to prepare for one event, such as a major exam or a massive project. If you like studying and working together, you can meet on a more permanent basis.

Your schedule is most likely to mesh with those of other students in your clinical rotation. See if you can interest a half dozen of them in joining you.

Successful study groups have certain ground rules. For the group to be effective, every nursing student in it must agree to the following:

Successful Study Groups

1. Understand and accept the purpose or mission.
2. Contribute ideas, information, opinions, and feelings.
3. Invite and encourage other members to do the same.
4. Listen intently.
5. Demonstrate respect and support for other members.
6. Help keep the discussion relevant.
7. Periodically help summarize the major points.
8. Give examples and share pertinent clinical experiences.
9. Recognize conflict and controversy as potentially positive, and refuse to see them as a personal rejection.
10. Refrain from eating, smoking, or *knitting* during the session.

How to Make a Good Study Group Better

TIME

Always meet at the same time.

PLACE

Always meet at the same place.

BEGIN

Always begin on time.

MONITOR

Appoint a monitor to keep the group on target and the discussion moving. Focus on the here and now. Don't let the group spend too much time dwelling in the past or fretting about the future.

GOAL

At the beginning of the session, state the goal. "Today we will discuss Chapters 4 and 5," or "This group is reviewing for the anatomy midterm."

DISCUSS

Allow free-flowing discussion of anything relevant to the group's goal. Identify major concepts, clarify discrepancies between text and lecture, share examples from clinical experience, and relate theory to practice. If questions arise that cannot be quickly and accurately answered, don't waste time pooling ignorance. Appoint one member to check with the instructor and report back to the group.

REVIEW

Review lecture notes, highlights of outside readings, films, class objectives, lists to be memorized, etc.

QUIZ

Drill each other. Use test questions at the end of the chapter or, better yet, construct your own.

"Lately we've each been bringing two trivia questions to group. Not only is it fun, it also forces each member to read and review before the study session. Constructing questions has helped me think the way instructors think when they're making up tests."

SUMMARIZE

Periodically pause and recap the major points under discussion. At the end of the session, summarize what you have accomplished and list the things that still need to be done.

DIVIDE

Whenever possible, divide tasks and activities.

"We split up the objectives, with each member being responsible for just a few. That person gathers the information and brings copies for everyone to the next meeting. It saves so much time!"

ASSIGN

Assign individuals or subgroups to tasks, and be sure to specify dates for completion.

END

Always end on time.

SOCIALIZE

After the official end of the group, members may feel free to leave or to stay and chat. The benefits of playing together should not be underestimated.

"We had a problem maintaining student morale, so about once a month we have some kind of a get-together where we can relax and talk or joke about our problems. Last semester we had 3 hours between classes, and every so often we'd order pizza to be brought in or we'd go out for lunch. At our Christmas party we all got together and composed a letter to Santa telling him about all our goofs in clinical. It was fun and reassuring to hear that everyone else made goofs like I did."

When students form study groups or support groups, they are "networking." You may be interested to learn that student networks reach far beyond your own campus. They operate on a national and an international level. If you would like to extend your network, write to:

National Student Nurses' Association
45 Main Street, Suite 606
Brooklyn, NY 11202
www.nsna.org
or
Canadian Nursing Students' Association
99 5th Avenue, Suite 15
Ottawa, Ontario, Canada K1S 5K4
www.cnsa.ca

Registered nurses band together in groups for the same reason students do—to survive. And for one even better reason—to thrive! If you would like more information about networks available for registered nurses, see Appendixes B through F for the names and addresses of major nursing associations.

Students helping students. Nurses helping nurses. That's a 10-4, Good Buddy.

CHAPTER 18

Preventive Maintenance

"Fatigue makes cowards of us all."
—Vince Lombardi

If you are a smart driver you know the value of preventive maintenance. You take simple actions to stop problems before they start. You know that by investing a few minutes, you can add years to the life of your car.

Every time you turn the key in the ignition, you should watch for warning lights on the dashboard. When you stop for gasoline, you should check the oil, water, and air pressure in the tires. Every few thousand miles, you should change the oil in your car, and after several thousand miles, you should replace the spark plugs and examine the fan belt for wear.

Self-Service

In fact, you may take better care of your car than you do of yourself. Those of us attracted to the helping professions are often good at taking care of everyone's needs but our own. We talk a lot about high-level wellness, stress management, and self-actualization, but few of us apply these concepts to our own lives.

We wouldn't run our machinery into the ground, but our personal motto seems to be "Don't stop till you drop." We don't even take time to fuel properly. We skip breakfast, eat lunch out of a vending machine, and drive through Burgers R Us for dinner.

Isn't it a pity that nursing students don't come equipped with instrument panels? Then you would know at a glance if your engine is overheating or your brake fluid is running low. Unfortunately you have no gauges, bells, whistles, or warning lights. Before you realize it, you may drive yourself right into a breakdown.

Preventive maintenance for humans is not as clear-cut as it is for vehicles. It probably includes things such as the following:

- Exercising regularly
- Reducing caffeine
- Avoiding unproductive stress
- Eliminating tobacco and alcohol
- Getting sufficient rest
- Taking vitamin supplements
- Keeping your sense of humor

The key words for a healthy lifestyle are *balance* and *moderation*.

When you find yourself under a lot of pressure and you need to talk things out, you may not be able to find a sympathetic ear. Instead of mumbling to yourself, it may be helpful to keep a written journal, a daily diary of everything that happens to you as a nursing student. For some reason, talking to yourself on paper is considered sophisticated. Talking to yourself out loud is considered schizophrenic.

Writing allows you to vent feelings safely, unscramble puzzling situations, explore new insights, and put events in perspective. Like a good friend, the journal "remembers" everything you've been through: all the firsts, all the good times, all the adventures and misadventures. On a bad day, when you forget how far you've come, the journal reminds you of your triumphs, not just your tragedies. The journal documents your growth. It chronicles not only your life and times but also the times of your life.

You can purchase an elegantly bound book full of blank pages or use a loose-leaf binder and ordinary notepaper. The journal is for your eyes only. There is no need to worry about spelling, punctuation, or grammar. You may worry about those things later if you decide to convert it to a bestseller.

Every so often, take a quick read of your daily journals. If the same problems and worries keep cropping up, you could be headed for depression. Researchers at the University of Michigan call it "rumination." Psychologist Susan Nolen-Hoeksema says women are prone to brood over problems instead of solving them and moving on with their lives.

Rumination may explain why women are twice as likely as men to fall victim to depression. Women experience more chronic strain than men, and they tend to feel less mastery and control over their lives. They ruminate. That aggravates the chronic strain, accentuates the lack of mastery and control, and increases the rumination. It's a vicious cycle. And the bad news is that bitching doesn't help.

What can you do? Watch yourself. Identify problems. Solve them. Don't get sucked into the downward spiral.

In the words of Mother Goose:

For every evil under the sun
There is a remedy or there's none.
If there is one, try and find it.
If there isn't, never mind it.

Being a nursing student can throw everything out of kilter. So pamper yourself. Have regular checkups. Use common sense. And WEAR SUPPORT HOSE! Remember, it is easier to prevent problems than to correct them.

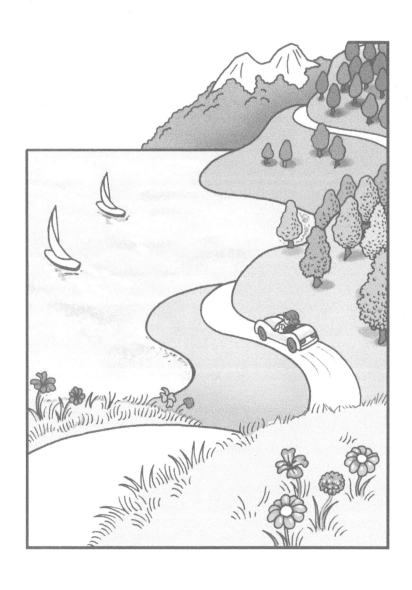

CHAPTER 19

Scenic Routes

"Life is a great big canvas, and you should throw all the paint on it you can."
—DANNY KAYE

As a nursing student you are usually compelled to go for speed and distance. The only chance you have to leave the main highway is through an occasional elective.

When it comes to choosing an elective, be sure to take the scenic route. Get as far away from nursing as possible. A brief excursion to some out-of-the-way discipline can be thoroughly refreshing and can help you return to the hard, fast pace of nursing with renewed energy and unusual insights.

Watch out for what former University of Rochester president Dennis O'Brien calls the "careerist syndrome." Having a rigid, narrow focus on career goals means missing exciting educational opportunities and graduating ill-equipped to deal with a fast-changing, increasingly complex world.

Once in a while you need a reminder that the whole world does not revolve around science or sickness. There are other worlds: art, music, drama, politics, economics, business, architecture...agriculture! Use your electives for field trips to these other worlds.

Nursing requires you to be so perfect and so practical that you may need an elective that allows you to be imperfect and impractical. Use electives for mental health breaks.

Because advisors are paid to look out for your future, they sometimes overlook your present. Consider your advisor's list of should-and-ought electives, then make your own choice. Instead of choosing an elective that will "expedite things in graduate school," choose one that will help you survive undergraduate school. Trust your instincts. You may be smarter to pass up intermediate statistics and opt for art appreciation.

If you have difficulty persuading your advisors to let you take offbeat electives, remind them that art, music, and drama all have therapeutic applications. Call on their interests in the legal, ethical, economic, or political ramifications of health care. Convince them that public relations is receiving as much attention from the hospital hierarchy as patient care. Confess that you have international (or even interplanetary) aspirations for nursing.

If all else fails, produce this ad, which appeared in a big-city newspaper:

Tell them that this is the job of your dreams and that you need this particular elective to improve your "sparkle" and "sense of humor." Sometimes an elective, just like this classified ad, brings much-needed comic relief. This ad shows that no elective should be deemed inappropriate.

Use the entire college catalog when you are searching for electives. Explore! Enjoy!

As you wander farther into nursing, you will be continually surprised by the variety of routes available. Some nurses enjoy caring for children; others enjoy caring for older adults. Some enjoy working in the emergency department; others enjoy working in intensive care, obstetrics, orthopedics, gastroenterology, or hospice nursing. If you thrive on delving into the subconscious, take the exit marked "Psychiatric Nursing." If you prefer the unconscious, take the "Operating Room" exit. You may veer off toward school nursing, occupational health nursing, or even private practice. The number of available routes will delight and confuse you.

How do you know which route will be right for you? While you are in school you will have several chances to sample different routes. Take full advantage of this opportunity. Push yourself to explore as many alternatives as possible.

When I taught at the University of Wisconsin–Madison, clinical experience in psychiatric nursing was an option, not a requirement. The students I had in this class were exceptional. Did they sign up because they thought they had an affinity for psychiatric nursing? No. Most of them were scared. They didn't have to come, and many confessed they didn't want to come, but they chose to come rather than miss a unique opportunity. All were glad they made the trip, even though only a few went on to become psychiatric nurses.

Instead of looking for an easy out or sliding along the path of least resistance, challenge yourself. Cultivate your adventurous streak. Be brave. Boldly go where no nursing student has gone before!

CHAPTER 20

Bridges

"Everything that irritates us about others can lead us to an understanding of ourselves."
—CARL JUNG

ourage. That's what I titled a piece of artwork I produced about the first black person to graduate from nursing school. Under a drawing of her I wrote these words: "Few of us are brave enough to be the first. Mary Eliza Mahoney was. As America's first black professional nurse she graduated from the New England Hospital for Women and Children on August 1, 1879. Mahoney was a first. A trailblazer. She didn't make it easy for others to follow but she did make it possible."

Someone always has to be the first. You may be the first person in your family to go to college. That makes you a trailblazer, too.

By enrolling in nursing school you have taken the first step on a bridge to another life. Nursing is a bridge from a dead-end job to a professional career. It is also a bridge from poverty to the middle class.

It doesn't matter whether you are red or yellow or black or white, if you are coming to nursing from the poverty class you are going to have challenges students from the middle class or the wealthy class won't have to face.

The most obvious one is a lack of resources. The good news is there is so much interest in making nursing more diverse, that a wealth of scholarships, loans, and stipends is available to minority or disadvantaged students.

Lack of a sound educational background is another problem. Students from the poverty class drop out of high school at alarming rates. Those students who do complete high school or get their GED, struggle in college. Many take assorted courses but never finish any degree.

The personal lives of those in the poverty class are often chaotic and disorganized. They have little idea how to set goals, establish priorities, or manage time. People from the poverty class live in the present, giving little thought to the past or the future. Time is to be enjoyed. Money is to be spent. Entertainment is highly valued. Unfortunately, "Eat, drink, and be merry" is not a motto that will help you succeed in nursing school.

Another trait of the poverty class is the belief in luck or fate. Either you are smart or you are not. End of story. These students give up easily and when the going gets tough, they quit. Let's be honest, the going in nursing school is always tough. As I wrote in that piece about Mary Mahoney, she broke ground that made it possible for others to follow. She did not make it easy. No one can make it easy.

You have to want nursing more than anything else. You have to dig up the money, carve out the time, sit in the classes, write the papers, take the tests, and often put food, drink, and fun on hold. You need to ask for help. And, you need to accept help when it is offered.

Get Out and Push

Although minorities comprise about 35% of our country's population, they comprise less then 12% of our profession's population. Nursing wants to look more like America, so the push is on to recruit more minority students. Who is a minority student? When it comes to nursing, it's anyone who is not a white female.

Are you man enough to be a nurse? Well, are you? These words were emblazoned on the hottest selling T-shirt at a National Student Nurses' Association convention. Fifty years ago only 4% of nurses were men. Today it's about 6%.

A statistic used to shame nursing about its lack of men is the fact that medical school enrollment has reached the 50/50 male/female mix. A former president of the Assembly of Men in Nursing said, "Nursing no longer has the luxury of accepting only females." *Luxury?* Necessity. What he failed to note is that while women have been clamoring to get into medicine, men have not been clamoring to get into nursing.

Men are one of the minorities nursing schools are vigorously recruiting and with notable success. In some schools men comprise 20% of the class. However, men, like other minorities, *drop out at twice the rate of majority students.*

What happens if you find yourself the only male student? Black student? Hispanic student? You may relish being unique or you may feel lonely, excluded, and alienated.

Connect with the Assembly of Men in Nursing, the National Black Nurses Association, or the National Association of Hispanic Nurses. If you can't find a mentor on campus, you may be able to find one online. Check out journals like *Minority Nurse*, the *Journal of Transcultural Nursing*, or the *Journal of Cultural Diversity*.

Role models and mentors can make a world of difference. Some colleges have big brother/big sister programs that pair advanced minority students with beginners. Minority staff nurses may be paired with students. Not only do they provide a realistic view of what nurses do, they are also living proof that success is within reach. Faculty are often assigned one or two students that they will mentor throughout the entire program. Unfortunately, minority faculty members are few and far between. Less than 11% of full-time faculty are minorities. Minority nurses interested in teaching will find all sorts of money available to help them get advanced degrees.

One college hired a recruiter who was very successful at attracting minority students. The college, however, was not very successful at keeping them, so they added a retention specialist to the staff. They found retention depends on getting specific help to the student in need.

For example, pre-nursing courses can be indispensable in helping students increase their proficiency in English, math, and science. Because many are single parents, they need more than scholarships, they need stipends so they can work fewer hours. They may need help with housing, transportation, or childcare. They need access to emergency funds. They need the flexibility of online courses and weekend programs. They need help with time management, critical thinking, test-taking skills, and stress reduction. They need supportive peers, staff, faculty, and family if they are to successfully complete the program.

Nursing is investing a lot of time, money, and effort into attracting and hanging on to these higher-risk students. Why? Because they have as much to teach us as they have to learn from us. As they share their stories, traditions, customs, dreams, and ideas, we learn how to provide better care to all our patients and communities. These students have great potential to become tomorrow's leaders. They will become the mentors and role models for future travelers on this road to nursing.

I was once asked to speak at a midyear commencement for an accelerated program of second-degree students at NYU. All were getting either their bachelor's or master's degrees in nursing. It was like addressing the United Nations. I have never stood before a class so diverse. The energy, the excitement, and the hope for the future of nursing that class embodied took my breath away.

Open Road

When you hit the open road to nursing, the best thing you can bring along is an open mind. You will be caring for, and working with, people of every race, religion, creed, culture, sex, sexual orientation, age, education, and income bracket.

To increase your flexibility and tolerance, exercise. Stretch yourself to the limits. Test your values. Examine their origins, their accuracy, and their usefulness.

Each of us is unique. Hispanics don't want to be lumped together any more than blacks, whites, or Asians do. Try as I might I will never really know what it's like to be black, or male, or Jewish, or gay, or dyslexic, or left-handed, or skinny. Try as I might, I will never know what it is like to be you. And you will never know what it is like to be me.

There will always be prejudice. There will always be a pecking order. There will always be stereotypes. You cannot let any of this distract you or deter you from your goal of becoming a nurse.

Nurses are supposed to be nonjudgmental—a noble concept that is impossible to attain. You will be judgmental. You will judge everyone on the basis of your standards, just as I will judge everyone on the basis of mine.

To keep judgmental attitudes from interfering with professional performance, you have to know yourself inside and out. Take a few moments to describe yourself by answering the following questions:

Age?
Sex?
Race?
Ethnic background?
Region of country?
Urban or rural?
Fat or thin?
Religion? How religious?
Political preference? How political?
Education?
Income level?
Pet peeves?
Favorite charities?
Energy level?
Optimistic or pessimistic?
Shy or bold?
Recreational pastimes or hobbies?
Dreams?
Fears?
Family commitments?

The more answers you have in common with someone, the more comfortable you will be with that person. Unfortunately, you cannot choose your patients, colleagues, or classmates as you do your friends. You have to take what you get and then work at establishing a relationship. The operative word is *work*.

Lillian Wald founded the Visiting Nurse Service back in the 1890s. The motto was "Response to every call for help without regard to race or creed or color." She coined the phrase "public health." She said, "People are either fed or hungry, warm or cold, well or sick, happy or unhappy." To her those were the only differences that mattered. We should follow her lead.

Taking Sides

On the highway there is always a right side and a wrong side of the road. In nursing, as in life, the distinctions are not that clear-cut. Every day you will deal with sensitive people and emotionally charged issues. You need to be fully aware of your attitudes on abortion, euthanasia, pain control, venereal disease, suicide, disability, disfigurement, abuse, addiction, and the right to die—to name only a few.

When you find yourself holding views diametrically opposed to those of your patients, classmates, teachers, or coworkers, it is difficult to keep from being offended or from offending others. Knowing your feelings is crucial because attitudes guide actions.

In nursing you need to be able to tolerate a great deal of ambiguity. You have to learn to live with choices that are not yours to make.

Strive to recognize differences as differences. Steer clear of the impulse to label them as right or wrong. You can't live happily in nursing until you understand that your way is only one way. There will always be alternate routes. Whenever you can, build a bridge.

CHAPTER **21**

Business Routes

"It has made me like working to see that writing is not a performance but a generosity."
—Brenda Ueland, *If You Want to Write*

When you are a student, your business is to deliver words on demand. Whether drafting a term paper, giving a report to the next shift, persuading an instructor to modify an assignment, writing a care plan, presenting an award, making a report to classmates, teaching a patient self-care, or addressing an international meeting, it all boils down to words.

When you need to get down to business, there are two routes you can follow. You can either deliver words in person, or you can deliver words on paper.

Words Delivered in Person

When you have to deliver words in person, the first rule is to know your audience. Will there be 1 person or 100? Regular people or professionals? Male or female? Age? Education? Primary interests? Familiarity with the subject? The better you know your audience, the better your chances for a successful presentation.

Next you have to know the purpose of your presentation. Are you supposed to stimulate interest, provide information, arouse to action, teach a skill, or entertain?

Consider how much time you have for your presentation. The amount of preparation time required for a good presentation is inversely proportional to the amount of time allotted. That means it takes more preparation time to give a good 10-minute talk than a good 60-minute talk. The less time you have to deliver your presentation, the more efficiently focused, tightly organized, and highly polished you have to be.

When you try to tell your audience "everything," they usually leave with nothing. Good presenters know how important it is to define and limit content.

To prioritize content, ask yourself, "If the audience could take away only one idea or piece of information, what should it be?" That becomes your first and foremost objective. What is the second most important idea for them to grasp? The third?

By prioritizing your content, you will know how much time and attention to devote to each section. And if you are allotted less time for your presentation than expected, you will know where to trim it without doing major damage.

THE CONSTRUCTION

Taking the three vital objectives you have identified, draft a bare-bones outline. Do whatever reading, research, or interviewing is necessary to flesh it out.

Some students prefer to write out their speeches word for word. That is fine if you promise not to read it word for word. Never, ever read your speech. You will bore people to death. Never, ever memorize your speech. You will bore yourself to death.

After you've constructed a comprehensive outline or drafted your entire speech, grab a couple of index cards. Now reduce your entire speech to a dozen key words or phrases.

THE REHEARSAL

Pick up your index cards and begin rehearsing. Play with alternate words and phrases. Then, when you stand before the audience, you will not suffer a loss for words or panic when you cannot remember the exact words.

Using a tape recorder during rehearsal is an excellent idea. Listening to yourself for the first time is often a shock. It may not sound like you to you, but that is the way you sound to others. Listen to your voice. Is it lively, well modulated, clear? Do you mumble, stammer, say "you know" 539 times? Check the pacing and your choice of words.

Resist the compulsion to fill every second with words such as "ah...uh... ahummm." Clearing your throat and coughing are usually nervous attempts to fill empty spaces. Actually, pauses and silences can have a powerful impact. With practice, you can learn to be comfortably quiet between thoughts.

Choose words that are positive. Make no apologies or excuses such as, "I wish I had had more time to prepare" or "You probably know more about this subject than I do."

Do not talk down to your audience. Do not snow them with statistics or use half your time dropping names of experts. Steer clear of slang, jargon, and profanity.

Consciously curb nervous gestures such as twisting your hair, pulling your ears, blinking rapidly, giggling, playing with your notes, or jingling the change in your pocket.

Sometimes it helps to rehearse in front of a mirror. Then you can see yourself as others see you. This shock may be even greater than the one you get from listening to yourself on the tape recorder. But if you are serious about improving your speaking skills, you have to be willing to critique yourself. Poise will come with practice.

When you rehearse, go through your entire speech from start to finish. If you make a mistake or forget an important point, make a graceful recovery and keep going. You won't be able to start over from the beginning when you face a live audience.

You also need to time yourself during rehearsal. Inexperienced speakers invariably underestimate the amount of time it takes for delivery. With 2 minutes left, half of their content remains untouched. Remember, nothing makes an audience happier than a speaker who ends on time, unless it is a speaker who ends 5 minutes early.

Have a full dress rehearsal, especially if you plan to wear new clothes or shoes. Test drive your outfit so you know your shoes won't pinch, your skirt won't ride up, and you can reach the top of the chalkboard without splitting a seam. Choose something that is comfortable yet attractive and very professional looking.

Are you a little nervous about your presentation? Good. A bit of anxiety gets the adrenaline flowing and helps you do your best. An overdose of anxiety, however, can paralyze you.

THE COUNTDOWN

There are several things you can do to keep anxiety under control. For example, visit the room where you will give your presentation. Check out the lighting, acoustics, exits, seating arrangements, the location of the nearest bathroom. Stand behind the lectern. Run through a few lines.

Decide where you will place any equipment or props. Practice using projectors or other mechanical devices.

If possible, mingle with the audience before your session begins. Introduce yourself, chat, eavesdrop. Learning a few names and faces can put things on a much friendlier basis.

If your throat is dry, take a sip of warm drink. Ironically, speakers are usually given a pitcher of ice water. A cold drink will contract throat muscles, but a warm one will relax them.

THE DELIVERY

Take a deep breath. Concentrate on the audience, not on yourself. Make eye contact. Smile. Even if there are 300 people in the room, speak to one person at a time.

Engage your audience as much as possible. Draw them in and get them to nod in agreement with what you are saying.

Although you should never memorize your whole speech, there are two parts you should memorize: your opening line and your closing line. Knowing exactly how you will launch your speech will reduce anxiety. Knowing how you can bring your speech to an effective close lets you be more relaxed and responsive during your speech.

Be sensitive to your audience. Do not ignore their needs by hurrying through your speech. Watch them. If they seem confused, bored, overheated, or agitated, stop. Find out where the problem lies. You may need to open a window, close a door, take an unscheduled stretch break, give them an individual exercise, or allow them to make comments and ask questions.

If you are giving a presentation to your classmates and you have only one picture, chart, or model, do not pass it around the group while you are talking. It is too distracting. Either make a copy for everyone, convert the material to a slide, or offer to make it available after the session for anyone who wants a closer look.

Audiovisual aids make a presentation more interesting and enhance learning. Pictures are literally worth a thousand words. The audience will forget 90% of your words but will remember pictures and the ideas behind them.

Handouts can supplement information and reduce the need for note taking. If you are only going to discuss three aspects of cerebral palsy, you may want to make a list of "20 Facts About Cerebral Palsy" with a suggested reading list. Participants like to have something in hand that they can take home.

If someone asks a question and you don't know the answer, say, "I don't know the answer, but I will have it for you tomorrow." If you make a mistake, admit it. If someone challenges your information, be ready to cite sources. If he or she persists, offer to meet later to compare and contrast information. If someone is argumentative, don't become defensive. Say, "That is a very interesting point of view. I would like to continue this discussion when there is more time."

Words Delivered on Paper

When you have to deliver words on paper, you can follow many of the same principles that apply to delivering words in person. First, know your audience. Who is going to read this paper? Write for the reader.

Decide on the purpose of the paper. Are you attempting to inform, persuade, or entertain?

Consider the importance of the assignment. Is this a daily exercise or a paper that will constitute half of your grade? The amount of time you invest should be proportional to the amount of benefit you expect to receive.

Next, choose a topic. Choosing is not as difficult as narrowing that topic down to a manageable size. Before you begin writing "Communicable Diseases Through the Ages" (a topic that would fill 10 volumes), talk to your instructor. You will probably end up writing something more like "Measles from 1910 to 1920." If you follow your instructor's advice and suggestions, success is almost guaranteed because your instructor is your reader.

Once you and your instructor have agreed on the topic, draft a brief outline. Then head for the library and the librarian. Librarians will direct you not only to current guides for nursing literature but also computer services that can generate a list of all relevant articles published in the last few years. The fee is nominal and well worth it if your time is short.

Usually your problem will be identifying quality articles. Occasionally the problem is finding an adequate number of articles. Several years ago I attended a meeting of the American Association for the Advancement of Science. One of the sessions, "The Oldest Old," was to focus on people older than the age of 85 (the fastest-growing segment of the population). When the sociologists who did the presentation went to the library to do research, they found nothing there. The subject was too recent. Today the amount of information available is absolutely overwhelming.

Provided what you need is in print, your librarian can help you find it. Even if your school is small and your library is limited, the librarian can arrange interlibrary loans. Books and journals can be sent from major health science libraries.

I had been working on a children's book about Lillian Wald, a turn-of-the-20th-century New York nurse who developed the Visiting Nurse Service, created the occupation of school nurse, and built one of the very first public playgrounds. I found that only a dozen books had been written on Wald, and I bought all of them online. I also bought the only two books she had written. Now, if you are a book collector, vintage books can be very expensive. But if you are a reader or researcher, you can get a perfectly usable book for a couple of bucks. The online bookseller saved me untold hours of time and made my research thoroughly enjoyable.

Before you spend much time reading any book or article, scan it. Titles are often misleading, and many that appear relevant are not.

As you read, watch for recurring themes, major issues, milestones, facts, and figures. Take notes on index cards. Keep track of questions that need answering.

Before you begin writing, refine your outline. Reorganize it and make it as comprehensive as possible. Decide which information carries the most weight. Prioritize objectives just as you did when you prepared your speech. What is the most important idea or piece of information? The second most important? The third?

FLOOR IT

Let your fingers fly when you write the first draft. Pay no attention to spelling, punctuation, phrasing, or logic. Scribble thoughts as fast as they occur to you. Whether you write or type, leave wide margins and plenty of space between lines where you can rewrite or add information.

Set the paper aside. Sleep on it. The next morning, work it over. Edit, reorganize, expand. Strive for simple words and short sentences.

Write a second draft. If possible, let 2 or 3 days elapse, then work it over again. Reading your paper aloud is often helpful.

Sometimes when you work long and hard on a project, you cannot see its fatal flaws. Let a friend check your paper for readability, logic, and content. Ask for a double check on spelling and punctuation. If you have a word-processing program with a spell checker, be sure to use it.

Just remember, even spell checkers have limitations. Here's a little ditty that made the rounds on the Internet:

ODE TO A SPELL CHECKER

I have a spelling checker,
It came with my P.C.;
It plainly marks four my revue,
Mistakes I cannot sea.

I've run this poem threw it,
I'm sure your please too no;
Its letter perfect in it's weigh,
My checker tolled me sew.

Formats for footnotes and bibliographies are varied. What is in vogue at one school will be inappropriate at another. Ask your instructor for guidelines. In an emergency, just follow the format in one of your recommended textbooks. As long as you are consistent in the way you handle references, you will not lose more than a couple of points.

When you print the final draft, use good-quality white paper (at least 20-pound, preferably with rag content). Make sure each page has a number and your name. Do a professional quality job on the title page and the cover. Neatness does count.

Finally, the only thing better than delivering your paper on time is delivering it ahead of schedule.

No matter what route you take after nursing school, skills as a speaker and writer will always help you.

CHAPTER 22

Hot-Wired

"The illiterate of the 21st century will not be those who cannot read or write, but those who cannot learn, unlearn, and relearn."
—ALVIN TOFFLER

Before you set foot in a school of nursing, you need a computer, preferably a laptop because of its portability, and you need to know how to use it. Oh, the places you will go…online.

Today "hitting the books" means hitting a computer key and having access to libraries around the world. Classrooms are equipped with wireless Internet access. Schools and faculty put their calendars, requirements, and course materials online. You can take classroom notes on your laptop, e-mail your term papers and care plans, and even take tests online. In the hospital you can download the latest information on drugs, diseases, and treatments. You suddenly have the freedom and flexibility to work from home—or the beach! You can log on at noon or at midnight.

Maria locked her keys in the car on a Friday afternoon, the last day of the semester. She was frantic because she was going to miss a class in which she was required to turn in her final paper. While waiting for the locksmith, she e-mailed her paper to the professor, telling him what had happened. That way he would know that she hadn't skipped school because she hadn't done her homework.

Instead of driving to a study group, you and your classmates can all log on and have a threaded discussion. If you have a question about an assignment or wonder where a test is being given, you can find out without playing telephone tag.

Websites like Facebook let you keep in touch with friends and family in a fun, fast, inexpensive way. The Internet lets you keep in touch with people around the globe. I was once invited to speak to a group of nurses in Japan. Two of my former classmates with nursing connections there went with me for a 10-day junket. In addition to sightseeing, we toured nursing schools, hospitals, and health care organizations in several cities. Today we can keep in touch with our newfound colleagues and friends via e-mail. It's quick. It's free. And, you don't have to worry about time zones.

Start Your Engines...Your Search Engines

The Internet can save you a lot of time and energy. You can check movie listings, compare auto prices, buy airline tickets, print out IRS tax forms, do a job search, check the weather around the world, find your best friend from kindergarten, tour an art museum in France, order office supplies, play the stock market, read an encyclopedia, or get a map with step-by-step directions to any address in any city.

The Internet can help you in hundreds of ways. For example, if you are having difficulty hearing the differences in heartbeats, google Auscultation Assistant, which lets you hear and practice identifying a variety of heart defects. Can't afford every reference book? If writing isn't your strong suit, go to The Purdue Online Writing Lab (www.owl.english. edu), the world's first online writing lab. It provides resources as well as online help.

The downside is that the Internet can also help you waste an enormous amount of time. Easily distracted people can spend hours wandering around cyberspace. For some it is as addictive as drugs, alcohol, nicotine, or chocolate! (Remember the chapter on detours?)

Don't Give Your Car Keys to Thieves

Crooks and thieves seem to be the first to master new technology. So only use your credit cards on secure sites, never reveal passwords or personal identification numbers (PINs), and don't give out your Social Security number.

Any product's greatest strength is also its greatest weakness. The Internet is rife with uses and abuses because it offers speed, open access, the illusion of anonymity, and a lack of geographic boundaries.

Scams abound. The Federal Trade Commission (FTC) is finding it difficult to keep fraudulent health products off the Web. Any advertisement that includes phrases such as "scientific breakthrough," "secret ingredient," or "ancient remedy" is suspect. Other clues include undocumented case histories or testimonials of "miracle cures" and claims that the government or the medical profession has conspired to keep this product from consumers. Another red flag is any product that is available from only one source. The FTC's home page has more advice on how to evaluate diet, health, and fitness products (www.ftc.gov).

Site Seeing

If you are writing a term paper and need a specific fact, the Internet can deliver it in a fraction of a second. In the same length of time, the Internet can overwhelm you with more information than you could use in a lifetime.

Using the search engine, Google, I just typed in "cancer," and in 0.06 second I found there were 10,900,000 entries containing that word. When I typed in "breast cancer," I found 1,720,000 entries. For "breast cancer support groups," there were 324,000 entries; for "breast cancer support groups in Iowa," there were 10,400 entries; for "breast cancer support groups in Des Moines, Iowa," there were 1100 entries. As you can see, the more specific you are in the key words you choose, the less material you will have to sift through.

It's hard to believe that in 1993 there were only 130 websites. Today there are millions. Every school, organization, agency, business, and bozo has a website.

Thousands upon thousands of sites are dedicated to health. How do you know which sites provide accurate, reliable, ethical, and useful information? It is not always easy.

First, consider the source. Check to see if the website is operated by a medical school, a teaching hospital, a government agency, a well-known consumer organization, an established support group, or a reputable professional. The site should provide the names and credentials of its authors and researchers. You can do a quick search to see if these "world-class experts" have published anything in legitimate professional journals. The site should tell you when it was last updated and should provide links to other compatible websites. Be aware that drug companies, equipment manufacturers, and the like have a vested interest. They will tout their own products and publish "scientific work" only if it improves their bottom line.

An outstanding website is www.healthfinder.gov, where you will find a wide variety of health topics selected from 1600 government and nonprofit organizations. The site offers personal health tools, helps locate doctors and health centers, and features the latest health news. Known for reliability, credibility, and excellence in health communication, this website is on the Medical Library Association's "Top 10 Most Useful Websites."

The top ten are chosen by MLA's Consumer and Patient Health Information Section. Websites are evaluated for credibility, sponsorship/authorship, content, audience, currency, disclosure, purpose, links, design, interactivity, and disclaimers. The other nine on that list are:

www.cancer.gov
Centers for Disease Control and Prevention (cdc.gov)
www.familydoctor.org
HIV Insite (www.hivinsite.ucsf.edu)

www.kidshealth.org

www.mayoclinic.com

MEDEM: an information partnership of medical societies (www.medem. com/medlib)

www.medlinePlus.gov (English or Spanish)

NOAH: New York Online Access to Health (www.noah-health.org)

Here are some other websites you may find helpful:

Agency for Healthcare Research and Quality (AHRQ). www.ahcpr.gov

American Diabetes Association. www.diabetes.org

American Heart Association. www.americanheart.org

Food and Drug Administration. www.fda.gov

Health On the Net Foundation. www.hon.ch

MEDLINE plus. www.medlineplus.gov

Medscape. www.medscape.com

National Institutes of Health (NIH). www.nih.gov

U.S. Department of Health & Human Services. www.hhs.gov

U.S. National Library of Medicine. www.nlm.nih.gov

WebMD. www.webmd.com

World Health Organization. www.who.int

It's wonderful to have access to the Library of Medicine, but you will not find the full text for many of the articles. You will primarily find abstracts—brief summaries—but that will be enough to tell you whether the article is worth tracking down. If you can't find the actual book or journal in your college library, you can get it through interlibrary loan.

Some online professional journals are free, but others have subscription fees just as printed journals do. The Internet lets you access articles from newspapers and popular magazines. There may be a small fee ($2 to $3) if you want to print it out. You can put it on your credit card.

Websites such as Medscape are free but require registration before you are given access. Medscape offers more than 100 medical journals, online continuing education, and daily medical news. Talk about a bargain!

Get your classmates involved in sharing their favorite websites. Make your own directory. Keep it current. Websites tend to appear and disappear with little rhyme or reason.

It Bytes!

Feeling invisible and anonymous, people visit places on the Internet they wouldn't dare go in real life. They think that if they just hit the delete button, no one will ever know where they went, what they did, or what they said. They think their actions will vanish without a trace into thin air. Wrong.

We've all seen the FBI confiscating the computers of suspected criminals, potential terrorists, sleazy businessmen, and mischievous teenage hackers on the evening news. The authorities can reconstruct all your activities just as they did with the medical student who became known as the Craig's List killer.

If you visit bad neighborhoods, you better expect trouble. So don't visit pornography or hate group sites. Don't gamble, perpetrate hoaxes, participate in get-rich-quick schemes, pose nude, make racial slurs, or pass along obscene jokes.

Some students have purchased term papers online and submitted them as their own. Maybe I should say "former students." It is not just lazy; it is unethical. It may get you kicked out of college or cost you your scholarship.

A University of Virginia physics professor, Louis A. Bloomfield, wrote a software program that compared student papers. He was able to identify 122 students who had copied paragraphs or entire papers from those of previous students and submitted them as their own. They were high-tech cheaters who were caught with high-tech methods. Poetic justice.

Whiplash

The Internet offers unparalleled opportunities and unprecedented problems for patients. They come to their doctors' appointments with printouts of information about the disease, fatality rates, standard medications, and experimental treatments. Many are not informed, they are misinformed. Part of your professional responsibility will be helping them differentiate rumors from facts and doctors from quacks. (You may want to refer them to www.quackwatch.com.)

Patients know they can order every conceivable drug online at bargain prices without a prescription. Whether the drugs are real or fake, pure or contaminated, helpful or harmful is anybody's guess.

On a more positive note, the Internet allows people to join support groups. Medical experts can talk the talk, but patients want first-hand information from experienced fellow sufferers and their families. Support group members lend sympathetic ears, dispense no-nonsense advice, and offer prayers, suggestions, and recommendations. When a message is sent out, even in the middle of the night, someone in the group will respond. It's always daylight somewhere in the world, and support groups span the globe! Patients say the biggest comfort is knowing that they are not alone and not crazy.

Speaking of crazy, you've heard of hypochondriacs. Have you heard of cyberchondriacs? A recent study by Microsoft researchers suggests people who use search engines to diagnose themselves usually conclude the worst. For them, headaches become brain tumors. A muscle twitch becomes Lou Gehrig's disease. Their anxiety goes through the roof.

Don't be surprised if you develop a few symptoms of your own. Most students do.

CHAPTER 23

In the Driver's Seat

"Experience is the name everyone gives to his mistakes."
—OSCAR WILDE

A few feet off the interstate, the exit split into northbound and south-bound lanes. The driver ahead of me was obviously unsure which lane was the "right" lane. Before he could make up his mind, he impaled his car on the lane divider.

If he had it to do over again, I am sure he would agree that even the "wrong" decision would have been better than no decision. He may have had to drive a little out of his way, but he would have arrived in one piece.

In a moving vehicle, decision time is limited. To be a good driver you need a ready mind and a steady hand. You need to size up situations quickly, make decisions, and take action.

The same is true of nursing.

When you are in the driver's seat you take full responsibility for your actions. When you make an error you must take the consequences. Even if some backseat driver gave you a bum steer, the citation will be issued to you.

The same is true of nursing.

Professionally speaking, when you are in the driver's seat, you take full responsibility for your actions. When you make an error, and you will, do not waste time making excuses. Face up to your responsibility. Learn from the experience. Then drive on.

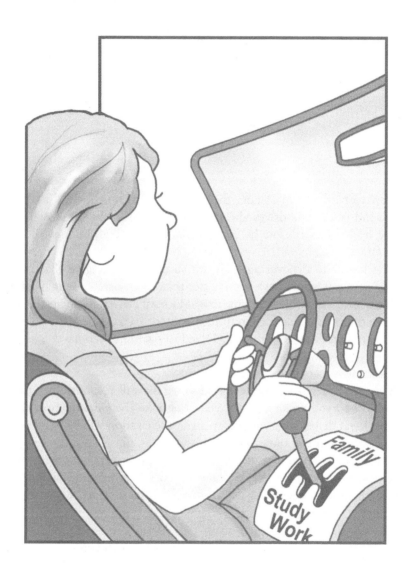

CHAPTER **24**

Shifting Gears

*"We are here on earth to do good for others. What the others are here for,
I don't know."*
—W. H. AUDEN

Going back to school after several years' absence can be a real jolt to the system. The song goes, "I will never pass this way again," and yet here you are back in school at 25, 30, 40, or 50 years of age.

Consider what happened to my sister. She is a business whiz. When a golden opportunity appeared, she did not see the need to finish college. She signed on with a rapidly expanding company and, through a combination of sheer talent and incredibly hard work, rose to a vice-president's position. She was on the fast track and confident that she had it made. Until her company merged. She found herself out on the street with several other top-level managers.

She quickly discovered that it was impossible to get a comparable position without proper academic credentials. Oh, there were jobs available but not the career opportunities she wanted. For example, one representative told her his company would not even interview her for a secretarial position without a bachelor's degree. She soon found herself back in school—a little older, a little wiser.

People who find themselves back in school at midlife are called "mature" students. Whether this is a first career venture, a move to enhance career options, or a complete career change makes little difference. In addition to the academic challenge, there are a multitude of other stressors.

Vintage Vehicle

Mature students don't worry about a date for homecoming. They worry about coming home and finding that the babysitter has quit, the cupboard is bare, the toilet is overflowing, the dog is in heat, and the mortgage is due. Meeting obligations means continually making tough choices and uncomfortable compromises.

137

Many mature students have to commute. They can't relocate their families, so they "dislocate" themselves.

"I was a full-time student at the university with a husband 200 miles away who claimed he couldn't cook for himself. I drove 200 miles on Friday to cook, clean, be the ideal wife on Saturday and Sunday. I drove back Sunday evening and spent the whole night studying for the week. Both grades and marriage came out intact, but I was physically and mentally exhausted."

A long drive to and from school can be a grueling experience. Here is how one student came to enjoy her roadwork.

"I spend 12 hours away from home at least 5 days a week. My 'spare time' is spent driving 2 hours each day to and from school. At first I resented the drive. Now I love it. I can sing all four parts to the choir songs. I love to listen to the news and the games. I recognize certain cars and trucks; we honk and wave, and I share a common bond with their drivers. Life has so many perks if you just look for them. My 2 hours behind the wheel have become a gift instead of a burden."

Maintaining a positive attitude and accepting the drive as part of the price of higher education will make the road seem shorter. Don't waste time and energy resenting reality. Go with it.

The road to nursing always goes uphill. If you want to make it to the top, you have to shift to a lower gear and lighten your load as much as possible. This is especially true for married students and those with children, regardless of age.

Married men have an advantage. They have wives. Married women have a disadvantage. They are wives.

Being a wife-mother-student means going into overdrive. After spending all day in class and clinical, you race home (driven by guilt), toss in a load of laundry, start dinner, vacuum the living room, balance the checkbook, check the kids' homework, walk the dog, and listen to an instant replay of your husband's day at work. When you finally get everyone bedded down for the night, you tiptoe to the kitchen table, spread out your books, and study until past midnight. The next morning you wake up tired and already behind schedule.

Many women fail to make the grade in nursing school because they refuse to lighten their loads. They vow that nothing will change. They try valiantly to do everything just as before, but they fall farther and farther behind. Women drive themselves too hard.

THEY'VE FOUND SOMETHING THAT CAN DO THE WORK OF 10 MEN...

Participants at a midwestern nursing management conference included approximately 100 women and only 1 man. All held demanding jobs in middle and upper management. The afternoon session dealt with the Superwoman complex—the compulsion to do everything perfectly, from cooking to cleaning to parenting to advancing a career.

The man, who was still a bachelor, was amazed at what he heard. He didn't see how the women could manage to do everything at work and everything at home. It had never occurred to him that he should do his own housework. As soon as he was employed, he had hired someone to come in twice a week.

It doesn't occur to men to do their own housework. It doesn't occur to women not to do their own housework. Time to shift!

After that conference, many of those nurse-managers probably hired housekeeping help. As a student you may not be able to afford help, yet you cannot afford to be without it. If you can't hire it, you have to commandeer it.

Just as it never occurred to the male manager to do his own housework, it will probably never occur to your husband to do his own housework. Studies show that husbands of working wives do no more household chores than husbands of nonworking wives. Chances are that this holds true for children, too. If you want your family's help around the house, you will have to be the one who says so.

Make lists of essential household chores, and let family members choose which ones they prefer to do. Divide the ones nobody wants and assign them on a rotating basis. Have some chores available for extra credit. These pay bonuses over allowances.

DANCING IN THE DUST

An Iowa student found that she could get the whole family to pitch in for 1 hour every Saturday morning. They turned on rock-and-roll music, and all six of them danced through the house doing their assigned chores.

If dancing house cleaners don't measure up to your exacting standards, relax your standards. In fact, if you are going to survive nursing school, you have to relax, period.

Family members can feel threatened as your friends, interests, lifestyle, and priorities shift. There may be some anger, fear, jealousy, and resentment. There can also be new joy, pride, fun, and adventure.

WHO IS THIS PERSON?

Nursing absorbs so much time and attention that one man complained that he had to make an appointment just to see his wife. A lot of the romance and spontaneity seemed to have gone out of their relationship. Their solution? They stopped thinking of their times together as "appointments" and began thinking of them as "dates." It revitalized their marriage.

The spouse always plays a critical role in the student's success or failure.

"As a diploma nurse the push is to get a degree and move on to a master's. When I was married with three children and a full-time job, I started back to school. My husband was very nonsupportive. 'That is more time away from me and the children.' I felt guilty about that, too, but I was also angry. I had supported my husband through his last year of college and 4 years of postgraduate work. I went ahead with school but eventually dropped out. I guess the guilt and nonsupport weakened me. I'm now divorced with a full-time job, three children, less money, and going to school because my job requires a bachelor's."

How supportive is your spouse?

NO SUPPORT   FULL SUPPORT

☐ ☐

Be honest. Support is not just talk: It's ACTION! As a student prepared to head for the library one evening, her husband groaned, "Do I have to babysit again?" She snapped back, "No, you don't have to babysit. The only children here tonight will be yours!"

When long-established patterns are disrupted, when standard operating procedures are violated, tensions mount and tempers flare. In many ways the whole family goes back to school. Everyone is learning, adjusting, and adapting.

As you return to school, it's nice to have the support of friends and family. Not every student is that fortunate.

"Upon deciding I wanted a career—not just a job—I pledged to give it my all. My parents and relatives did not understand. My husband has always been supportive, but comments from those 'outside' our lives really hurt. They would say things like 'You sure are neglecting your husband' or "It's too bad you can't spend more time together' or 'You can do that; you don't have children.' I decided to set my own goals and do what was needed to attain them. I have been successful. Whether other people support me or not, I made the decision that this is MY life and I'm doing these things for ME!"

How important is it for you to have the approval of family and friends? Can you stand alone? Can you say with this student, "This is *my* life and I'm doing these things for *me*"? If you can, your chances of success are much greater.

KIDDIE CARE

The more support you have from your children, the better your chances of surviving nursing school. Let them know that things will be different. Help your family make the shift.

Involve your children as soon as possible and as much as possible. Talk to them about your school. Take them to the library, your classroom, the nursing skills laboratory, and the hospital. Children are much more comfortable when they can visualize where their parents are.

Make nurse kits for your children. Toss in syringes, tongue blades, bandages, finger cots—whatever you can scrounge. Buy them a stethoscope of their own.

One family had "study hall" around the dining room table from 7:00 to 8:30 PM. Another family had each member go to a separate room and close the door for a "quiet hour."

To survive you need a private place where you can study. Privacy is something mothers are not supposed to need. Moms are supposed to be accessible 24 hours a day, 7 days a week, 365 days a year. Shift!

Go to your room. Close your door for 1 hour. Let an older child or your spouse handle problems and answer questions. When you emerge from study time, be ready to give your full, undivided attention to the family. If they know you will be really available at a certain time, they will permit you a study hour.

Even though you can't do everything together, you can do the important things together. What are the most important things? Ask your child, "What's one thing you would like us to do together today?" It may be having a special story read, hosting a tea party in the tree house, shopping for new tennis shoes, going to the zoo, working on a school project, or playing Monopoly. Let your children help plan special evenings, weekend outings, or vacation events.

Recognize that although you can do anything, you cannot do everything. You have to make choices.

For example, while driving across the country one summer, we decided to take a 200-mile detour and spend one day in a city where we had lived for several years. How could we see everyone in just 24 hours? We couldn't. So each of us chose the one person we most wanted to see. When we entered the city limits, we phoned the four people and made arrangements to see them.

Then we drove to our old neighborhood and fit in other people and activities as we could. We left bright and early the next morning, feeling very satisfied and happy that we had made the detour.

Women Drivers

One of the most popular workshops I teach is designed for women who are trying to do it all, have it all, and be it all. I call it "Walk-On-Water Women" (WOW for short). I ask participants to describe a situation in which two or more of their roles are in conflict. Many of the examples involve women who are back in school and trying to be good wives, good mothers, good daughters, good neighbors, good employees, and good students *simultaneously!* It is exhausting.

In her fascinating book, *Sequencing,* Arlene Rossen Cardozo talks about women who have chosen to do it all, but not simultaneously. These women have had the foresight or the fortitude or the good fortune to have completed their education, established themselves firmly in careers, and then chosen to experience full-time mothering. I would call this sequencing with a capital "S." And I personally know of only one woman who has managed to pull this off.

For the rest of us—the frantic, the frazzled—who are trying to do it all simultaneously, I would like to recommend sequencing with a small "s." It begins with acknowledging that you cannot be in two places at once.

"Sometimes I feel torn—I'm working and in school, and on weekends I need to clean house, do laundry, scrub floors, cut grass, etc., etc., etc. My husband wants to do something fun for the weekend. I feel the need to spend time with him and the family, but then I have twice as much work to do when I return home—tired kids, dirty laundry, messy house. Most of the time I give in and then pay the price later for the fun. But again, sometimes I don't enjoy myself much because I know what's waiting for me when I get home—and return to work and school the next day! Sometimes I resent my husband for not being able to see the work that needs to be done at home."

Here is another student with the same conflict but a much healthier way of handling it:

"When do I feel stressed? When behind in classes and housework and needing to do a million things at home! Like last Saturday when hubby and kids wanted to go to the cottage for a day but I didn't—I wanted to get caught up. This caused a conflict between my needs and theirs. After a 'discussion' the family went without me. I got everything done and felt good about the day. They came home having had a great day, and we wondered why we had argued."

In nursing school your social life will be sharply curtailed. With little time for family, you will have almost no time for friends. Say goodbye to dinner parties and hello to potlucks. You can also invite friends over just for dessert, or you can have a taco party to which everyone brings his or her favorite ingredient. True friends don't come for the food; they come for the fun of being together, and true friends won't mind if your house was cleaned by six rock-and-roll dancers.

Socialize with your classmates and their families. Families can compare notes, swap stories, sympathize with each other, and help solve problems.

Always have contingency plans. If the babysitter falls through, who is the backup person? If one of the children is sick, who will stay home? If the car breaks down, what alternate transportation is available? Contingency plans include a spare house key hidden in the flower pot, a spare lasagna in the freezer, a spare $20 bill under the mattress, and a spare uniform in the closet. Then you can shift at a moment's notice.

Professional Drivers

Whether male or female, young or old, you have to be able to shift gears when you enter the hospital. You must switch to your professional gear. For instance, people two or three times your age will be asking you for advice. They will tell you things they wouldn't tell their best friend, their spouse, or their clergy. You must respect these confidences, always protecting your patients' privacy and dignity.

With some practice, shifting from the personal to the professional mode becomes almost automatic. There are times, however, when that shift must be a conscious, deliberate decision.

For example, one nurse had some nagging personal problems that began interfering with her ability to concentrate at work. One day she noticed a large laundry basket parked outside the operating room area. As she passed by, she decided to dump her personal problems mentally into that basket. At the end of her shift, she mentally picked up her personal problems. Turning her personal life off during working hours made her happier and more productive. After work, even though she "picked up" her problems again, she felt better able to carry them. She approached her personal life with a new freshness and was able to resolve her problems in a short time.

Making the Grade

Mature students are often more uptight about grades than their younger counterparts. They feel driven to excel. Perhaps it is one way to justify all the time, energy, and money being diverted into school. Perhaps mature students want to set a good example for their own children. Whatever their motivation, they don't want to be good students—they want to be great.

Grades can become more important than learning. I know it's true. I've been there. I have spent a major portion of my life as a student. I feel like the fellow who quipped, "I've been in school so long I know things that just ain't so."

Like other overachievers, I have my own private grading system. If I get an A, I'm not always sure I earned it. I know I could have done more, learned more. If I get a B, I'm upset because Suzie-Q got an A, and I know I'm just as smart and worked just as hard as she did. If I get a C, I'm destroyed. For a highly competitive person like me, that's an automatic failure.

When I approached graduate school, I wanted things to be different. First of all, I wanted to combine psychiatric and pediatric nursing, but no such program existed. I devised one of my own. I took electives, did extra reading, and arranged my clinical assignments to reflect my private agenda. While conforming on the surface, below the surface I was busily doing my own thing.

I knew that if I let my grades influence me, I would neglect my own priorities. So I chose not to know my grades. To receive your grades at the University of Washington, you had to turn in a set of stamped, self-addressed envelopes. I didn't turn in any envelopes. I did not see my grades the entire time I was in graduate school. I figured if I were in academic trouble, someone would tap me on the shoulder and tell me to shape up. If I were doing OK, then it was just that—OK! The pursuit of perfection wouldn't sidetrack me.

During my fourth quarter I discovered what a liberating experience it had been. Evidently, one faculty member was a notoriously unfair grader. My fellow students were up in arms, ready to get tar and feathers. I just smiled to myself. I didn't know my grade. It honestly didn't matter to me. I had learned what I wanted to learn and had already moved on to other things.

Sometimes the only way to get where YOU really want to go is to shift gears and "brake" with old habits and traditions. Do whatever it takes to make sure learning is more important than grading.

Buying American or Japanese?

When educational psychologists gave an unsolvable math problem to groups of Japanese and American children, they uncovered one key as to why our academic achievement is so much lower. The American kids struggled briefly and then gave up. The Japanese kids kept working, apparently believing that if you persist you can solve any problem.

Hard work is the key to success. Yet many Americans believe the key to success is inborn talent. Either you have it or you don't. Educational psychologists say our obsession with natural talent and innate ability has produced kids who give up easily. In fact, many Americans believe people who work hard in school must lack ability.

If you believe people are born smart, chances are you're a quitter. If you believe people are made smart, you'll knuckle down, persevere, and succeed! You'll know what Thomas Edison knew—that genius is 1% inspiration and 99% perspiration.

Being able to shift gears quickly is essential if you are to survive nursing school. From now on, you will have to shift more; "shiftless" students won't make it.

CHAPTER 25

Moving Violations

"Anyone who has never made a mistake has never tried anything new."
—ALBERT EINSTEIN

The summer before I went to nursing school, I worked a couple of months as a nurses' aide. I received no training or orientation. I was dumped directly onto a busy floor during the evening shift. The nurse in charge would teach me the ropes as she had time.

I ran errands, fetched water, delivered dinner trays, and was assigned to help patients get ready for bed, which included giving backrubs. The charge nurse told me to use lotion and powder.

My first "victim" was Maxine, a patient quite debilitated with multiple sclerosis. I smeared lotion all over her broad back and then liberally sprinkled powder on top. The two ingredients combined to form a lumpy paste. The more I rubbed, the worse it got.

Maxine shrieked, "Good grief, girl, what do you think you're doing!" I replied, "Making pie crust." She burst into laughter.

I explained it was my first night, and I really had no idea of what I was doing. Immediately she became my teacher. I learned a lot of basics from Maxine, including how tough it is to be a patient. She wrote to me while I was a nursing student, and whenever I got home, I went to see her. She died shortly after I graduated.

Fortunately you won't be tossed into the hospital in such a casual way. Before you hit the road, you will receive a lot of instruction.

Most of us had a driver's education course, and before we were allowed on the road, we spent hours reading, studying, and testing. There were films, demonstrations, discussions, and simulators to approximate driving conditions so that we could rehearse responses to all sorts of situations. When we passed the first part of the course, we were allowed to get behind the wheel of a specially equipped car. At our side sat an instructor using a dual-control system to keep us from making any dangerous errors. After we passed written and driving exams, our licenses were granted. For the first time we were allowed to drive solo.

Nursing education follows much the same pattern. Before you are allowed to touch a patient, you spend hours reading, studying, testing, and rehearsing all sorts of technical procedures. If you are successful in the nursing skills laboratory, an instructor will accompany you to the patient for a real test of your ability. The instructor is there to protect you and your patient from any serious error. If you pass the patient test, you are allowed to do the procedure solo.

Being able to pass the "patient test" is crucial. If you fail the clinical portion of the course, you fail the course. There is no grade averaging here. Even straight-A students who fail clinical are out. The course must be repeated.

Mastering the skills and procedures of nursing practice is essential. To survive in nursing you must be able to use your hands as well as your head.

Of the students who botch the clinical component, only one in a thousand is a complete klutz. The others are usually ill-prepared or experience acute anxiety attacks that interfere with their performance.

To be prepared you need to make the most of your time in the nursing skills lab. While waiting for your turn, you can learn a lot from your classmates. Keep alert. Watch every movement. Listen to the instructor's comments and the responses of your classmates. Envision yourself in your classmates' place. Feel the equipment in your hand. Anticipate each step. Recite the rationale to yourself. Concentrate.

Using Your Head

Sports experiments have repeatedly confirmed the value of "synthetic" experience. For example, in a classic study, students were divided into three groups and then tested on their ability to shoot free throws. For almost 3 weeks after the initial testing, group 1 practiced shooting free throws, group 2 did nothing related to basketball, and group 3 spent 20 minutes every day imagining they were shooting free throws. At the final test, group 2 showed no improvement, but groups 1 and 3 improved 24% and 23%, respectively. Studies like this one indicate that the human nervous system cannot distinguish between an actual experience and a vividly imagined one.

PICTURE PERFECT

If you picture yourself failing, you double your chances of failure. If you picture yourself succeeding, you double your chances of success. So picture yourself doing the procedure and doing it perfectly, with precision and finesse. Mentally rehearse.

To control your anxiety, take slow, deep breaths. Focus on the patient and his or her needs. Recognize that sweaty palms, cold feet, butterflies in the stomach, and lightheadedness are normal symptoms of anxiety. Once the procedure is complete, they will disappear.

Be assured that you will never be permitted to perform a procedure on a patient that you haven't perfected in the skills lab. Remember that the instructor will be right by your side to coach you and keep you from doing harm.

The first time you perform any procedure is nerve-racking at best. Some students keep trying to postpone the inevitable. They keep their heads down and stand at the back of the group, hoping they won't be chosen. Although it is possible to get through nursing school with minimum experience, it is not possible to get through with no experience.

Every time you postpone doing a procedure, anxiety builds until it reaches panic proportions. Confidence is the only cure, and confidence comes from competence. Competence comes from experience, and experience often comes the hard way. So keep your head up, stand at the front of the group, and volunteer.

I asked nurses what they would suggest students do to help take the terror out of clinical experience. Here is what they said:

"Remember that you are a student and there to learn. So ask questions and don't be afraid of not being perfect."

"Take a deep breath and say, I'm OK! I can do it!"

"Believe in yourself. Don't sweat the small stuff!"

"Don't ever be afraid to ask how to do something or admit you don't know an answer. We've all been in your shoes."

"We were all students once—remind us of what it's like. Ask for help and guidance."

"Don't tell the patient this is your first time. It isn't. You've practiced this over and over in the classroom."

"Just put yourself in the patient's place and think about how you would like to be treated."

"Relax. Be calm. The patient is a person just like you."

"Determine what will REALISTICALLY happen if you goof or screw up. The patient won't die and neither will you."

"Blow the situation so out of proportion that you'll laugh. Picture yourself and the patient as cartoon characters."

"Remember every nurse from the director of nursing on down had to take this first step."

"Don't let your instructor intimidate you. Remember, she was once a terrified student like you."

"Actually, your instructor wants you to pass/excel even more than you do. Think about it! If you don't look good, she doesn't look good. She's cheering for you."

"Pray."

"The first time is always terrifying. Go on—do it! The second time it feels better and works better."

"Realize anyone can make a mistake. There is no such thing as a bad experience. Always look for the positive. What have I learned from this?"

"Don't be afraid or embarrassed to try. Even if you blunder, remember that doing is learning. It leads to confidence. Grab every experience you can!"

To get adequate experience, you may not only need to volunteer, you may have to fight to volunteer. Time in the clinical area is limited, and the procedures available are at a premium. You may get only one opportunity to perform a certain procedure. Once is not enough to build confidence or competence. To get more than minimum experience, make sure the staff knows which procedures you need to practice and which ones you are allowed to do solo. Make sure they know you are ready, willing, and able.

In driving and in nursing, the most serious infractions are moving violations. To keep from being labeled "unsafe at any speed," practice, practice, practice.

CHAPTER 26

Defensive Driving

"In law a man is guilty when he violates the rights of others. In ethics he is guilty if he only thinks of doing so."
—IMMANUEL KANT

W hen you drive defensively, you protect yourself by watching out for the other guy. In many ways, watching out for the other guy is the very essence of nursing. Caring for and about others is our business. We have traditionally been more concerned about the rights of others than about our own rights.

Delineating "the other guy's" rights has become a national pastime. Every conceivable group has a "bill of rights." Patients have several champions. For example, here is the American Hospital Association's version of a patient's bill of rights. It was first adopted in 1973 and last revised in 2003.

The Patient Care Partnership: Understanding Expectations, Rights, and Responsibilities

When you need hospital care, your doctor and the nurses and other professionals at our hospital are committed to working with you and your family to meet your health care needs. Our dedicated doctors and staff serve the community in all its ethnic, religious, and economic diversity. Our goal is for you and your family to have the same care and attention we would want for our families and ourselves.

The sections explain some of the basics about how you can expect to be treated during your hospital stay. They also cover what we will need from you to care for you better. If you have questions at any time, please ask them. Unasked or unanswered questions can add to the stress of being in the hospital. Your comfort and confidence in your care are very important to us.

What to Expect During Your Hospital Stay

High-quality Hospital Care. Our first priority is to provide you the care you need when you need it, with skill, compassion, and respect. Tell your caregivers if you have concerns about your care or if you have pain. You

Continued

The Patient Care Partnership: Understanding Expectations, Rights, and Responsibilities—cont'd

have the right to know the identity of doctors, nurses, and others involved in your care, and you have the right to know when they are students, residents, or other trainees.

A Clean and Safe Environment. Our hospital works hard to keep you safe. We use special policies and procedures to avoid mistakes in your care and keep you free from abuse or neglect. If anything unexpected and significant happens during your hospital stay, you will be told what happened, and any resulting changes in your care will be discussed with you.

Involvement in Your Care. You and your doctor often make decisions about your care before you go to the hospital. Other times, especially in emergencies, those decisions are made during your hospital stay. When decision making takes place, it should include:

Discussing your medical condition and information about medically appropriate treatment choices. To make informed decisions with your doctor, you need to understand:

- The benefits and risks of each treatment
- Whether your treatment is experimental or part of a research study
- What you can reasonably expect from your treatment and any long-term effects it might have on your quality of life
- What you and your family will need to do after you leave the hospital
- The financial consequences of using uncovered services or out-of-network providers

Please tell your caregivers if you need more information about treatment choices.

Discussing your treatment plan. When you enter the hospital, you sign a general consent to treatment. In some cases, such as surgery or experimental treatment, you may be asked to confirm in writing that you understand what is planned and agree to it. This process protects your right to consent to or refuse a treatment. Your doctor will explain the medical consequences of refusing recommended treatment. It also protects your right to decide if you want to participate in a research study.

Getting information from you. Your caregivers need complete and correct information about your health and coverage so that they can make good decisions about your care. That includes:

- Past illnesses, surgeries or hospital stays
- Past allergic reactions
- Any medicines or dietary supplements (such as vitamins and herbs) that you are taking
- Any network or admission requirements under your health plan

Understanding your health care goals and values. You may have health care goals and values or spiritual beliefs that are important to your well-being. They will be taken into account as much as possible through-out your hospital stay. Make sure your doctor, your family, and your care team know your wishes.

Understanding who should make decisions when you cannot. If you have signed a health care power of attorney stating who should speak for you if you become unable to make health care decisions for yourself, or a "living will" or "advance directive" that states your wishes about end-of-life care, give copies to your doctor, your family, and your care team. If you or your family need help making difficult decisions, counselors, chaplains, and others are available to help.

Protection of Your Privacy. We respect the confidentiality of your rela-tionship with your doctor and other caregivers, and the sensitive informa-tion about your health and health care that are part of that relationship. State and federal laws and hospital operating policies protect the privacy of your medical information. You will receive a Notice of Privacy Practices that describes the ways that we use, disclose, and safeguard patient information and that explains how you can obtain a copy of information from our records about your care.

Preparing You and Your Family for When You Leave the Hospital. Your doctor works with hospital staff and professionals in your community. You and your family also play an important role in your care. The success of your treatment often 'depends on your efforts to follow medication, diet, and therapy plans. Your family may need to help care for you at home.

You can expect us to help you identify sources of follow-up care and to let you know if our hospital has a financial interest in any referrals. As long as you agree that we can share information about your care with them, we will coordinate our activities with your caregivers outside the hospital. You can also expect to receive information and, when possible, training about the self-care you will need when you go home.

Help with Your Bill and Filing Insurance Claims. Our staff will file claims for you with health care insurers or other programs such as Medi-care and Medicaid. They also will help your doctor with needed documen-tation. Hospital bills and insurance coverage are often confusing. If you have questions about your bill, contact our business office. If you need help understanding your insurance coverage or health plan, start with your insurance company or health benefits manager. If you do not have health coverage, we will try to help you and your family find financial help or make other arrangements. We need your help with collecting needed information and other requirements to obtain coverage or assistance.

While you are here, you will receive more detailed notices about some of the rights you have as a hospital patient and how to exercise them. We are always interested in improving. If you have questions, comments, or concerns, please contact _____.

The Patient Care Partnership: Understanding Expectations, Rights and Responsibilities can be downloaded from www.aha.org in several languages including Arabic, Chinese, Russian, and Spanish.

In addition to general rights for general patients, all sorts of highly specialized subgroups have their own lists of rights: the disabled, the retarded, the pregnant, the dying, ad infinitum.

The American Nurses Association protects patients by spelling out nurses' responsibilities in a code of ethics, as shown here.

American Nurses Association Code of Ethics for Nurses

1. The nurse, in all professional relationships, practices with compassion and respect for the inherent dignity, worth and uniqueness of every individual, unrestricted by considerations of social or economic status, personal attributes, or the nature of health problems.
2. The nurse's primary commitment is to the patient, whether an individual, family, group, or community.
3. The nurse promotes, advocates for, and strives to protect the health, safety, and rights of the patient.
4. The nurse is responsible and accountable for individual nursing practice and determines the appropriate delegation of tasks consistent with the nurse's obligation to provide optimum patient care.
5. The nurse owes the same duties to self as to others, including the responsibility to preserve integrity and safety, to maintain competence, and to continue personal and professional growth.
6. The nurse participates in establishing, maintaining, and improving healthcare environments and conditions of employment conducive to the provision of quality health care and consistent with the values of the profession through individual and collective action.
7. The nurse participates in the advancement of the profession through contributions to practice, education, administration, and knowledge development.
8. The nurse collaborates with other health professionals and the public in promoting community, national, and international efforts to meet health needs.
9. The profession of nursing, as represented by associations and their members, is responsible for articulating nursing values, for maintaining the integrity of the profession and its practice, and for shaping social policy.

Nursing students have written their own code of conduct. Here it is.

National Student Nurses' Association Code of Academic and Clinical Conduct

Preamble

Students of nursing have a responsibility to society in learning the academic theory and clinical skills needed to provide nursing care. The clinical setting presents unique challenges and responsibilities while caring for human beings in a variety of health care environments.

The Code of Academic and Clinical Conduct is based on an understanding that to practice nursing as a student is an agreement to uphold the trust which society has placed in us. The statements of the Code provide guidance for the nursing student in the personal development of an ethical foundation and need not be limited strictly to the academic or clinical environment but can assist in the holistic development of the person.

A Code for Nursing Students

As students are involved in the clinical and academic environments we believe that ethical principles are a necessary guide to professional development. Therefore, within these environments we:

1. Advocate for the rights of all clients.
2. Maintain client confidentiality.
3. Take appropriate action to ensure the safety of clients, self, and others.
4. Provide care for the client in a timely, compassionate, and professional manner.
5. Communicate client care in a truthful, timely, and accurate manner.
6. Actively promote the highest level of moral and ethical principles and accept responsibility for our actions.
7. Promote excellence in nursing by encouraging lifelong learning and professional development.
8. Treat others with respect and promote an environment that respects human rights, values, and choice of cultural and spiritual beliefs.
9. Collaborate in every reasonable manner with the academic faculty and clinical staff to ensure the highest quality of client care.
10. Use every opportunity to improve faculty and clinical staff understanding of the learning needs of nursing students.
11. Encourage faculty, clinical staff, and peers to mentor nursing students.

Continued

National Student Nurses' Association Code of Academic and Clinical Conduct—cont'd

12. Refrain from performing any technique or procedure for which the student has not been adequately trained.
13. Refrain from any deliberate action or omission of care in the academic or clinical setting that creates unnecessary risk of injury to the client, self, or others.
14. Assist the staff nurse or preceptor in ensuring that there is full disclosure and that proper authorizations are obtained from clients regarding any form of treatment or research.
15. Abstain from the use of alcoholic beverages or any substances in the academic and clinical setting that impair judgment.
16. Strive to achieve and maintain an optimal level of personal health.
17. Support access to treatment and rehabilitation for students who are experiencing impairments related to substance abuse and mental or physical health issues.
18. Uphold school policies and regulations related to academic and clinical performance, reserving the right to challenge and critique rules and regulations as per school grievance policy.

Reprinted with permission from the National Student Nurses' Association, copyright 2001.

Nurses want to do more than conform to the letter of the law: we also want to conform to the spirit of the law. We take our responsibility for the rights of others very seriously.

As nurses we are so involved in protecting the rights of others that we often forget we have rights of our own. Perhaps that is why my list of "10 Basic Rights for Nurses in the Health Professions" attracts so much attention.

1. You have the right to be treated with respect.
2. You have the right to a reasonable workload.
3. You have the right to an equitable wage.
4. You have the right to determine your own priorities.
5. You have the right to ask for what you want.
6. You have the right to refuse without making excuses or feeling guilty.
7. You have the right to make mistakes and be responsible for them.
8. You have the right to give and receive information as a professional.
9. You have the right to act in the best interest of the patient.
10. You have the right to be human.

It is not the rights themselves, but the very idea that nurses have rights, that is novel.

As a nursing student you may be surprised to find that you have rights, too. For example, you have the right to see your educational records and to challenge information that you believe is inaccurate. Your records are to be kept private. With the exception of the registrar and your current instructor, no one should have access to your files without your permission. These rights are not at the discretion of the school but are legislated by Congress (Buckley Amendment). As expressed by the National Student Nurses' Association (NSNA):

"Every member of a nursing school must be held accountable for his/her action, be it an instructor, administrator or a student. NSNA believes that every school of nursing should have a written agreement between its students, faculty and administration."

This may be a good time to check into student rights on your campus. Rights are usually tucked away among the written rules, regulations, and requirements. They should include protection from capricious grading, incompetent instructors, and unsafe environments and should also provide specific guidelines for grievance procedures. To drive defensively you should know your rights long before you have to use them.

Even when rights are carefully spelled out, however, we know that there is a big difference between conforming to the letter of the law and conforming to the spirit of the law. Take the example of "informed consent." This is a paper that patients are asked to sign before surgery or treatment is undertaken. The document was developed to protect patients' rights. The intent was to make sure physicians instructed patients about their diagnoses, alternate treatments available, and potential risks or complications as well as potential benefits.

If you read consent forms from your local health care institutions, you will quickly see that they are written in terms only physicians and lawyers can understand. You will not be surprised to learn that (a) many patients think they have to sign and (b) the vast majority think the purpose is to protect physicians' rights, not their own.

By obtaining the patient's signature, the physician has "consent." He or she has conformed to the letter of the law. If the patient is truly "informed," then the physician has conformed to the spirit of the law as well.

Most of us want to live up to the spirit of the law. All of us have to live up to the letter of the law if we want to maintain licensure and avoid litigation.

Until recently nurses were seldom named as defendants in lawsuits. There were two reasons for this. First, nurses' salaries were so low that it literally did not pay to sue us. Second, nurses were assumed to be merely carrying out orders. We were not held accountable.

Today, nurses are named in lawsuits right along with doctors and hospitals because our salaries have risen substantially and because nurses now carry malpractice insurance. That makes them profitable targets. In addition, nurses are no longer seen as robots mechanically carrying out doctors' orders. The law perceives us as fully functioning professionals and holds us responsible for our actions and for our failure to act. In fact, the law requires nurses to exercise more judgment than some physicians, administrators, or nurses may deem acceptable.

The legal implications of nursing care are so complex that whole books are devoted to the subject. Professional journals frequently run articles dealing with legal issues in nursing, and many have regular columns on the subject. Law has become a popular graduate school option for nurses, and the number of nurse-attorneys is growing rapidly.

To avoid the courtroom you must take a road that is paved with paperwork: charting, care plans, anecdotal notes, incident reports, and discharge summaries. Although paperwork is time consuming, it should never be treated as trivial.

Donna Lee Guarriello, a nurse-attorney, provides a graphic illustration of the importance of paperwork. The case involved a young woman who had a cerebral hemorrhage and became permanently paralyzed after the birth of her first child. Initially, Guarriello intended to name the nurse together with two physicians in the lawsuit. After all, the nurse had spent 8 hours caring for the patient. During that time the patient's condition had steadily deteriorated. Apparently the nurse had been negligent.

After reading the nurse's notes, however, the attorney decided not to sue her. According to the chart, the nurse had repeatedly tried to get proper attention and treatment for the patient. She had phoned the attending physician, suggesting that he transfer the patient to intensive care. He refused. She contacted her supervisor. When the attending physician did not come to the hospital and did not return her subsequent phone calls, she arranged for another obstetrician and a resident to see the patient. Unfortunately, they refused to countermand the orders of the attending physician.

Everything was thoroughly, objectively, and professionally documented in the patient's chart. The nurse had not been negligent—quite the contrary. Paperwork did not help the patient, but it did save the nurse.

Always remember: Defensive driving begins and ends with paperwork. When it comes to documenting patient care, pay close attention to your instructor. Don't waste time complaining about the amount of paperwork involved in nursing. Learn to do it efficiently and effectively. Your professional life may depend on it.

CHAPTER **27**

Street Smart

"A positive attitude will not solve all your problems, but it will annoy enough people to make it worth the effort."
—JOHN GALSWORTHY

You are traveling through a tough neighborhood. People here are sick and angry. And that's just the faculty! You have the staff and patients to deal with, too. What a shame everyone seems to gang up on students. You would swear no one remembered what it was like to be the new kid on the block.

Don't they remember what it was like to be a student? Yes, they do. They remember exactly what it was like. Most went through hell and high water to become nurses. Many are still convinced that it is the only way to initiate you into the profession. Before you can be a member you have to prove your mettle. You have to show that you can stand up and take it like a nurse.

The only way to become part of any gang is to pay your dues. In nursing that means working together shoulder to shoulder, 40 hours a week, 50 weeks a year, for years and years. So when you enter the clinical setting, don't be surprised to feel like an outsider. You are an outsider. You are not part of the gang. If you are lucky, the staff will treat you like a guest. If you are unlucky, they will treat you like a trespasser.

Your instructor may or may not be part of the gang. Some faculty members have joint appointments, meaning they are employed by the educational as well as the health care institutions. They have real-life responsibilities for both the clinical unit and the classroom.

Most instructors, however, have a sole employer: the school. Consequently their status in the clinical unit may be almost equivalent to that of a student. Some instructors are warmly welcomed; others are barely tolerated. Given enough time and effort, faculty can earn a place in the gang. If your instructor has done so, count yourself lucky.

Nursing service and nursing education are often at odds. Each has a different mission, and sometimes they appear to be at cross purposes. Education strives for the ideal, whereas service must struggle with what is real.

For all practical purposes, you and your instructor are just passing through. The staff lives here. This is their turf, hard fought and hard won on a daily basis.

If you want to survive in this neighborhood, do not criticize the staff. Over the years you will learn that there is a big difference between being book smart and being street smart.

To pave the way for the best possible clinical experience, you not only need to give a good first impression, you also need to *get* a good first impression.

Getting a Good First Impression

Unfortunately every hospital is different, and every unit in every hospital is different. Just when you begin to feel comfortable in one clinical setting, you must rotate to another. Each new rotation begins with orientation—a rapid tour accompanied by a continuous stream of rules, regulations, policies, and preferences.

By the end of the tour some students are so anxious that they can no longer tell a crash cart from a laundry cart. Their senses are jammed by the sights, sounds, and smells of the unit. Instead of reducing their anxiety, orientation seems to accentuate it.

If orientation gives you a headache instead of a head start, you may want to make a preorientation visit to the facility and to the unit to which you are assigned. Many students recommend visiting your new clinical setting a few days early. To get a general feeling of the place, they suggest you sit in the lobby, spend time in the patient waiting areas, eat in the cafeteria, and just ride the elevators. Make a mental map of the way to your unit, the nursing office, the major departments, laboratories, and clinics. Students recommend visiting your specific unit during the evening shift because it is usually less hectic than the day shift. Whatever time of day you choose, you are cautioned to avoid change-of-shift periods.

Giving a Good First Impression

Make sure you arrive at the clinical unit clean, pressed, and appropriately dressed. Wear your name tag and look like you mean business. The more professional you look, the more professional courtesy will be extended to you.

Stand tall and walk confidently. Look people in the eye. Smile. Be energetic but not hyperactive. Control nervous gestures such as cracking your knuckles or twisting your hair.

Introduce yourself and ask for the person in charge. Give your name, rank, and serial number. State your purpose and ask permission to enter the unit.

"I'm Sherry Jackson, a second-year student, and I'll be in this unit beginning Monday. Would it be OK if I looked around a little? I'd like to get my bearings before orientation."

If you want to get along with the gang, always show respect for their territory and their time. Remember the staff nurses' names. Call them by the title they prefer. Be friendly. Be sincere.

Let the staff do most of the talking. Be a good listener. Encourage them to talk about themselves and their professional experiences. You can learn a lot vicariously.

Ask their advice. Respect their opinions. Avoid arguing, criticizing, or complaining.

Get them to reminisce about their student days. They have some wonderful tales to tell. Listening to their war stories will reassure you about the future. If they survived, so can you. Recalling their past may also make them more sensitive to your present needs.

Always be ready to do a little more than required. Volunteer to give a hand without being asked. Say please and thank you. Common courtesy is all too uncommon.

Patients Please

Often first impressions are formed even before you meet your patient. If you spend too much time studying the chart before going to his room, you may picture him as a series of problems, not as a person. If a staff member says, "So you're the one who got stuck with Mr. Elmers," you will have a much different first impression than if you are told, "Mr. Elmers is a terrific fellow. You are going to enjoy caring for him." Try to suspend judgment. Realize that first impressions or second-hand impressions may be more harmful than helpful.

The approaches that you used to make a good first impression on the staff can also help you make a good first impression on the patient—for example, dressing appropriately, looking professional, and controlling nervous gestures.

Before entering a patient's room, knock. Ask permission to enter. Respect what precious little turf the patient has.

Focus on the patient instead of on his tubes, dressings, or machinery. Look him in the eye. Pull up a chair and sit down. Introduce yourself and ask what name he prefers to be called. Tell him who you are and when you will be caring for him.

Before you leave, ask if he has any questions or if there is anything you can do for him. A simple act such as making sure the call bell is within reach, fetching fresh water, dialing the phone, fluffing the pillows, or finding out when he is scheduled for surgery can win him over.

Hearing with Your Eyes

Street-smart students know that body language often contradicts verbal language. A patient winces yet says, "I'm fine." The head nurse says, "Welcome to 4 West," but her arms are folded tightly across her chest and her body is rigid.

Learning to listen with your eyes as well as your ears helps you interpret what is happening more accurately. By studying nonverbal communication you will learn how to read people.

For example, did you know that leaning your head on one hand indicates interest, but leaning on both hands indicates boredom? Did you know that crossed arms are a sign of a closed mind, that locked ankles indicate worry or uncertainty, that a hand covering the mouth shows a lack of confidence and a reluctance to talk? Did you know that when people lie they tend to have rapid eye movements, lick their lips, rub their eyes, or scratch nervously?

As you learn more about body language, you will understand why it is not so much what you say but how you say it that counts. You observe one doctor who calls, "How are you?" from the doorway and another who goes to the bedside, touches the patient's shoulder, and asks the same question. The words are identical, but the effect is totally different. Which doctor really cares about the answer? Which doctor is going to get the more accurate response?

When trying to make a good impression, you choose your words carefully. Make the same careful choices when it comes to appearance, posture, and gestures. Actions do speak louder than words. Just ask any street-smart student.

CHAPTER 28

Life in the Fast Lane

"To succeed, jump as quickly at opportunities as you do at conclusions."
—BENJAMIN FRANKLIN

W ell, it's time for one last lap around the track. And the last lap may be the hardest. *"People told me each year got easier—not true! Each year is harder."*

If you are approaching your final year, you may appreciate these tips from students who were only days away from graduation. To prepare for that last go-round, they suggest you:

"Spend the summer reviewing everything you've covered."

"Get all nonessentials [anything that doesn't pertain to school] out of the way before entering that last year."

"Get a summer job in a hospital. That experience will help you make the most of your last year."

"Try to identify your niche in nursing and request clinical experience in that area."

At the beginning of your final year, most students say, "Really kick it into high gear" and "Give it all you've got!"

"Try to get every possible experience. Keep in mind how quickly a year goes. Get everything you can NOW!"

"Challenge yourself. Don't worry about grades."

"Keep your eye on your goal. Make every moment count."

"Quit your job. Don't work if at all possible. Focus all your energies on learning anything and everything."

"Read every nursing journal you can get your hands on."

"Join all the professional organizations and clubs you can."

"Attend in-service programs at the hospital whenever possible."

"Get involved. Become politically, financially, and professionally informed—do not have tunnel vision about your profession."

"Work hard...it will all be over soon."

Other students suggest you ease up a bit on the accelerator:

"Relax! This is what you've been waiting for. You're about to accomplish a very important goal."
"Enjoy your last year. When it's over, you're going to miss it."
"Relax. You know more than you think you do."
"Take time out to reflect on all you've accomplished."

No matter how tough things get, don't quit! A student from Texas said, "If I can make it, you can make it!" She's right. Every year about 120,000 nursing students "make it."

You might as well be one of them. So... ...

"Don't give up! Keep fighting!"
"Hang on!"
"Think POSITIVE!"
"Keep swimming, Babe, the shore is in sight!"

The good news is that you are about to graduate. That's also the bad news. If you graduate, you have to face state board examinations formally known as NCLEX-RN®. The mere mention of the final to end all finals—produces something akin to mass hysteria. These near-graduates suggest that you not become obsessed by state boards but rather prepare for them confidently and systematically.

"First things first. Concentrate on school."
"Write for information on state board testing dates."
"Buy a review book and pledge to spend 15 minutes a day with it."
"Form a group specifically to study for boards."
"Don't panic. Your instructors will help you. After all, if you don't look good, they don't look good."
"Enroll in a review course. They are available." (A list of Mosby's review books and courses appears in Appendix G)

As graduation approaches and attentions shift to finding a job, seniors advise you to:

"Start surveying employment opportunities early. Read the nursing career guides as well as the classified ads in newspapers."
"Form a job-search club. Critique each others' résumés. Discuss local and national career opportunities."
"Talk with recruiters and write to as many hospitals as possible for information. Photocopy anything you get, and share it with classmates. You're all in this together."

"Look for a mentor. See if there's an opportunity to work alongside a nurse you admire."

"Look for a hospital that offers an extensive, comprehensive internship program for new grads."

"Talk to last year's graduates and find out how they like their jobs. Ask them for suggestions. Is there anything they wish they had done differently in their senior year?"

"Remember, nursing is loaded with possibilities. Keep an open mind about specialization, new directions, and professional goals. You may be surprised!"

CHAPTER 29

Are We There Yet? Almost

"Double, double toil and trouble
Fire burn, and cauldron bubble
—WILLIAM SHAKESPEARE, *Macbeth*

Y ou have graduated from nursing school. Now the nightmare begins.

A tiny stretch of road is all that remains between you and your destination. But it winds through the dreaded NCLEX-RN®. (Cue diabolical laughter.) One last test. One last chance to totally screw up your life.

It's enough to make you scream…unless, you know the facts. In 2008 NCLEX-RN had 129,121 first-time takers and 86.7% passed. That same year 29,264 made a second attempt and 53.3% passed. The first quarter of 2009, the pass rate was 88%. So, even though it is possible for you to fail, it is not probable.

This is not a "Gotcha!" test brewed by some cauldron-stirring witches in a fiendish plot to dash all your hopes and dreams. It doesn't contain eye of newt, toe of frog, or wool of bat.

The NCLEX-RN is a carefully crafted, meticulously researched, and painstakingly refined test prepared by the National Council of State Boards of Nursing. The National Council Licensure Examination (NCLEX) has one purpose only: to determine if it is safe for you to begin practice as an entry-level nurse.

Entry-level nurse. Not expert-level nurse.

When I graduated from nursing school, "state boards" were given only twice a year in very limited locations. Hundreds upon hundreds of new graduates were herded into huge auditoriums where we spent 2 grueling days being tested.

Today the testing is much more humane. Instead of being herded into an auditorium far from home, you will make an appointment for a 6-hour time block at a testing center in your own community. You will sit in a carrel, take a short tutorial on how to use the computer, and then begin the exam.

You will answer between 75 and 265 questions. Each test is unique. That's because the test responds and adapts to the individual taking it. If you answer a question correctly, your next question will be a bit more difficult. If you answer incorrectly, your next question will be a bit easier. This enables the computer to calculate your level of competence.

The vast majority of the questions are multiple-choice but you may be asked to fill-in-the-blank, arrange a list in the right order, or place an X-marks-the-spot on a picture, diagram, or graph. You will be given an erasable white board to help you work things out, and you may use the computer's calculator.

You cannot change an answer once you have locked it in and you cannot skip a question.

While you were in nursing school, your tests measured your ability to recall and regurgitate. NCLEX is very different. You have to forget all the test-taking tips and clever strategies that got you through nursing school exams. They won't help you with NCLEX.

The focus of this last, best test is not on what you know. It is on what you are able to do with what you know. The unifying theme is "Meeting Client Needs." You must use your professional judgment to select answers that will provide safe, effective patient care. It's a test of your critical thinking, problem-solving, and decision-making abilities.

Like a good detective you will use your powers of observation to spot patterns and relationships. You will ask questions. In fact, you will question the question. You will reword and rephrase it to make sure you know exactly what is being asked. You will look for clues in the answers provided. You will use your knowledge of the normal to spot the abnormal. You will delineate the important from the urgent. You will beware of red herrings—information that distracts you from the true answer. You will make good use of what you have learned from anatomy, pharmacology, pathology, psychology, and nursing.

Each answer must be read as carefully as the question. There will be times when the answers all seem to be correct or incorrect. Don't panic, don't give up—think! Stay focused. You can often find the best answer by eliminating the other answers one by one. Remember to always give the "textbook" answer. The real world is ambiguous. The ideal world is not. NCLEX answers go strictly by the book.

NCLEX questions probe your ability to maintain and promote health while keeping clients intact physically, mentally, and emotionally. Your years in nursing school have given you a wealth of knowledge. You will use that knowledge to deal with advanced directives, case management, delegation, ethical practice, documentation, accident prevention, handling hazardous materials, asepsis, aging, family planning, newborn care, physical assessment, chemical dependency, crisis intervention, therapeutic communication, elimination, nutrition, palliative care, sleep, dosage calculations, diagnostic tests, laboratory values, vital signs, electrolyte imbalances, radiation therapy. And that is just the tip of the iceberg.

You will be asked to handle emergency situations (remember your ABCs: airway, breathing, circulation). You be asked to set priorities. For example, there may be a description of four patients. You will be asked which one would you attend to first? Or which one might you assign to a licensed practical nurse?

Over the years you have had the steps of the nursing process drummed into your head: assessment, analysis, planning, implementation, and evaluation of care. In school you used those steps to create patient care plans. Now those steps will help you solve the riddles of NCLEX.

Your school of nursing will help you through this final stretch. They will make sure you know how to register for NCLEX, certify your eligibility for the exam, and give you information on applying for licensure from your state board of nursing. You will most likely be given a "diagnostic test" to pinpoint your strengths and weaknesses. Faculty may offer review courses and study groups. Last year's successful test takers may share what they found most helpful.

Given the breadth, depth, and importance of this test, it is not surprising that you will spend between 3 weeks and 3 months preparing for the NCLEX-RN. An entire industry has sprung up to help you. You don't have to go to a health sciences bookstore. Go to any chain bookstore in your neighborhood and you will find shelves stuffed with books, workbooks, CDs, and flashcards all designed to help you pass this test. You can enroll in a commercial course designed specifically for NCLEX-RN. You can sign up for an online review course like the one offered on the National Council of State Boards of Nursing website.

Almost every review book includes a CD with test questions designed to mimic NCLEX-RN questions both in style and content. This is as close to a real-test simulation as you can get. By answering test questions on your own computer, you can immediately see what you got right and where you went wrong. Graduate nurses who passed the exam said that they answered 2000 or more practice questions. Some answered twice that many. By the time you get into that carrel on test day, you will be very comfortable with the format.

Away We Go!

Once you have graduated and passed the NCLEX-RN, you have arrived. And yet the journey is just beginning.

You surrender your learner's permit and pick up a professional license. One moment you are a thoroughly experienced student. The next moment you are a thoroughly inexperienced professional.

But if you have gotten this far, you can do anything!

CHAPTER 30

Kick the Tires and Light the Fires

"Your old life has crashed and burned; your new life isn't apparent yet. You may feel yourself to be temporarily without a vehicle. Just keep walking."
—JULIA CAMERON, *The Artist's Way*

First jobs are like first loves. The experience may be passionate but it is rarely permanent. That's why employers are often reluctant to hire new graduates. They know new grads are fragile and fickle. Fragile in that they need more support, guidance, time, and attention. Fickle in that they are full of romantic notions and will play the field, looking for the ideal job. When the going gets tough, they get gone. They head down the road looking for greener pastures.

If you feel fragile and fickle, you are not alone. New graduates are under a lot of pressure. While you were in school, there was always an escape clause. You could change your mind and your major. Now you have graduated. You are not going to be a nurse, you are one!

Graduation often brings elation followed quickly by depression. Not unusual—great achievement is often followed by a let-down. Your life has been so tightly structured, so highly goal directed, you have had no time to breathe. Until you can establish new patterns and set new goals, there is a void. Post-graduation blues are common, normal, and temporary. So relax.

Unfortunately school did not prepare you for work any more than courtship prepared you for marriage. Living with nursing day in and out, up close and personal, is different than visiting it three times a week. The honeymoon is over. The daily grind begins. The first year in any marriage or career is tough.

Getting a job is the next hurdle. For some of you making that first job decision is a done deal. You will be living and working in the same community where you went to school. Opportunities are specific and limited. Glamorous assignments in far-away places may call but you cannot answer. Your life is here. Be realistic. Don't torture yourself.

Get out an area map and mark off hospitals within a certain number of miles or minutes. If you are in a major metropolitan area, you may have 20 hospitals from which to choose. If you are in a small town, you may have only 1.

And the Winner is...You!

If you are footloose and fancy free, you will have more trouble making a decision. In a nurse shortage, jobs are plentiful everywhere. Pick the city of your choice. Before setting off to see the world, however, you may want to get a year of experience under your belt. It will be less stressful than simultaneously tackling a new job, a new career, and a new community.

In either case, the best way to approach this difficult decision is to take a piece of paper and split it into four quadrants. Label one half "Job A: Advantages and Disadvantages" and the other half "Job B: Advantages and Disadvantages." Fill in each section as best you can, then go in search of more information. Visit the facility, interview staff nurses, talk with last year's graduates, contact faculty for recommendations, eavesdrop in the cafeteria, see the nurse recruiter.

In any given community nursing salaries will be virtually the same. Only a few pennies per hour will separate one from another. Beware of any hospital offering bonuses or unusually high salaries by local standards. There is always a reason why they offer combat pay.

In fact, salary should be one of your last considerations in choosing a first job. You need to go where you can learn real-world nursing. You want to go where they provide an adequate orientation, a modified internship, access to mentors and preceptors, and nurse support groups.

Also consider which institutions offer whatever is most important to you. Each nurse has different needs and desires. What do you want most? Dental care, onsite childcare, tuition reimbursement, opportunities to specialize, an easy commute?

Narrow your selection down by playing one institution against another. Take the winner and compare it with the next challenger. If you get to a point at which you are torn between two seemingly equal opportunities, break the tie by flipping a coin. Flip a coin? Yes. Let me explain.

Heads or Tails?

Every nurse has come to a personal or professional crossroads and stood immobilized, terrified of making the wrong choice, the wrong decision. I've been there, too, and the most helpful piece of advice I can offer comes from Theodore Isaac Rubin's book *Overcoming Indecisiveness*.

Rubin says the big fact is that in very few situations does it actually make any difference which decision you make. (Whew! What a relief!) It doesn't matter whether you move to Florida or stay in Wisconsin, take the job in Med-Surg or in Psych, rent or buy, marry Fred or Charlie. You can be successful either way because success is not determined by which decision you make, it is determined by the level of commitment once the decision is made.

Rubin says very few people have the ability to pull out all stops, to commit wholeheartedly, 110%, and back their decisions to the hilt. If you can do that, you can make a success of almost anything.

If your experience is like mine, I have not yet faced a decision that did not have strong advantages and strong disadvantages on both sides. I think that lends credibility to Rubin's theory that you can be successful either way. Commitment will determine success.

When I suggested you flip a coin to break the deadlock between two jobs, I was not joking. It works. Every year I teach dozens of workshops with a decision-making focus. In one such workshop a nurse was trying to decide whether to stay in Denver or move to Seattle. After painstakingly identifying all the pros and cons, Jeanne was even more frustrated. She couldn't decide. I told her to bring me a quarter and I would tell her exactly what she should do.

As the two of us stood in front of 200 other nurses, I told her I was going to flip the coin. Heads she moved to Seattle. Tails she stayed in Denver. There was complete silence as the coin flip-flopped through the air. When it came up heads, I said, "Congratulations! You are moving to Seattle! How do you feel about that?" With barely a moment's hesitation, she shot back, "I'm so excited! I can hardly wait to get going!"

The audience burst into laughter. Of course, she didn't have to live by the flip of the coin. What was obvious to everyone including Jeanne, was that she could wholeheartedly commit. She could make a success of the move. In her heart of hearts she wanted to go.

If the color had drained from her face upon hearing "heads" or if she had physically backed away from me, sputtering a list of reasons why she shouldn't or couldn't move, we would have known that even if coerced into a move, she would sabotage herself. The move would be extremely stressful and probably not successful.

In another workshop I was dealing with nurse managers. Ruthann was struggling with whether to keep her job (she had a very good job) or open her own business. I told her to bring me a quarter. The coin toss said she should stay in her job. Before I could even get that complete sentence out of my mouth, her face fell. Her whole body slumped. She was so disappointed.

Time out for a reality check. Again, Ruthann did not have to live by the flip of a coin. What was obvious to everyone in the room was that she had already emotionally disengaged from her job. She was primed and ready to make a change.

If she did not follow her gut-level instincts she would probably always regret it. The unhappiest people in life are not the ones who saw opportunity, went out on a limb, and failed. They are the ones who saw opportunity and lacked the courage to go out on the limb after it. They continue to kick themselves, 20, 30, 40 years after the fact.

Once you decide on which job to take, commit completely—body, mind, and spirit. It is the key to success.

Enter the new job as you would a new class. This is where the real learning begins. Some employers and colleagues will expect you to hit the road running and be up to speed moments after graduation. You and I know that just does not happen. Although you have the basic knowledge you need, you lack street smarts. You are about to learn all the things they never taught you in nursing school. Welcome to Working Nurse 101!

Shake, Rattle, and Roll

The transition from student to practitioner is rigorous, so take special care of yourself. Keep your life as uncomplicated as possible. Make sure to get enough rest, eat right, and exercise.

Cut yourself some slack even when others don't. Instead of agonizing over what went wrong each day, take a moment and write down one or two of the good things that happened while you were on duty. Keep a diary. Track your progress. After 3 months, 6 months, a year, you will be so much more comfortable as a nurse. Have fun. Take up a sport or hobby. Reactivate your social life. Go where you want to go. Do what you want to do. There is so much more to life than your job.

Keep things light. One hospital unit experienced a horrendous turnover. It was now staffed almost entirely by new graduates. The head nurse helplessly watched them struggle. Morale was so low she thought they would not only leave her unit, but leave nursing.

During a particularly tense moment, as one new grad passed a panic-stricken colleague, she sang softly, "Don't Worry. Be Happy." That oldie-but-goodie song became their secret rallying cry. Within 30 days things had completely turned around. All the new grads made it. They didn't lose a one. The head nurse began to boast she had the best staff in the hospital.

So kick the tires and light the fires. Take your fragile, fickle, new graduate self and find the best possible job you can. Commit completely. Pamper yourself during the next few months. Keep your sense of humor. Stick together with your colleagues and "Don't Worry. Be Happy."

Appendixes

APPENDIX A

Common Prefixes and Suffixes Used in Nursing

PREFIXES	MEANING
a-, an-	without, not
ab-	away from
ad-	to, toward
adeno-	gland
aero-	air
ambi-	around
amphi-	about, on both sides, both
ampho-	both
ana-	up, back, again, excessive
angio-	vessel
ano-	anus
ante-	before, forward
anti-	against, counteracting
ap-, apo-	from, separation
arterio-	artery
arthro-	joint
bi-	double
bili-	bile
bio-	life
bis-	two
brachio-	arm
brady-	slow
broncho-	bronchus
cardio-	heart
cata-	down, under, lower, against
cepha-, cephalo-	head
cerebro-	cerebrum
cervico-	neck
chole-	gall, bile
cholecysto-	gallbladder
chondro-	cartilage
circum-	around
co-	together
com-, con-	with, together
contra-	opposite, against
costo-	ribs
cranio-	head
cyto-	cell
cysto-	bladder
de-	away from

PREFIXES	MEANING
demi-	half
derm-, derma-	skin
dia-	between, through, apart, across, completely
dis-	from
dorso-	back
dys	difficult, abnormal
e-, ex-, exo	out, away from
ec-	out from
ecto-	on outer side, situated on
electro-	related to electricity
em-, en-	in
encephal-	brain
endo-	within
entero-	intestines
epi-	upon, on
equi-	equal
eryth-	red
extra-	in addition to, outside of
ferro-	iron
fibro-	fiber
fore-	in front of, before
gastro-	stomach
glosso-	tongue
glyco-	sugar
hemi-	half
hemo-, hema-	blood
hepa-, hepato-	liver
histo-	tissue
homo-	same
hydro-	water
hyper-	high, excessive
hypo-	low, decreased
hyster-, hystero-	uterus
im-, in-	in, into, not
infra-	below
inter-	between
intra-	within
intro-	in, into, within
juxta-	near, close
laparo-	abdomen
laryngo-	larynx
latero-	side
leuk-	white

PREFIXES	MEANING
lympho-	lymph
macro-	large
mal-	poor, bad
mast, masto-	breast
medio-	middle
mega-	large, great
meno-	menses
meta-	beyond, after, change
micro-	small
mono-	single
multi-	many
myelo-	spinal cord, bone marrow
myo-	muscle
naso-	nose
neo-	new
nephro-	kidney
neuro-	nerve
nitro-	nitrogen
noct-	night
non-	not
ob-	in front of, against
oculo-	eye
odonto-	tooth
oophoro-	ovary
ophthalmo-	eye
opistho-	behind, backward
orchio-, orchido-	testes
ortho-	straight, normal
os-	mouth, bone
osteo-	bone
oto-	ear
ovario-	ovary
pan-	all
para-	beside, along with
path-	disease
ped-	child, foot
per-	by, through
peri-	around
pharyngo-	pharynx
phlebo-	vein
photo-	light
pneumo-	air, lungs
pod-	foot
poly-	many, much

PREFIXES	MEANING
post-	after, behind
pre-, pro-	before, in front of
proct-, procto-	rectum
pseudo-	false
psych-	mind
pyo-	pus
pyro-	fever
quadri-	four
radio-	radiation
re-	back, again
reno-	kidney
retro-	backward
rhino-	nose
sacro-	sacrum
sclero-	hard, hardening
semi-	half
spleno-	spleen
steno-	narrowing, construction
sterno-	sternum
sub-	under
super-, supra-	above, excess
sym-, syn-	together
tachy-	fast
teno-	tendon
thyro-	thyroid
trache-	trachea
trans-	throughout, across
tri-	three
ultra-	beyond
un-	not, reversal
uni-	one
uretero-	ureter
urethro-	urethra
uro-	urine
vaso-	blood vessel
veno-	vein

SUFFIXES	MEANING
-able	able to
-algia	pain
-cele	swelling, tumor
-centesis	surgical puncture
-cide	destructive, killing
-cule	little

SUFFIXES	**MEANING**
-cyte	cell
-ectasia	expansion, dilation
-ectomy	excision
-emia	blood
-esis	action
-form	shaped like
-genesis	origin, formation
-graph	writing
-iasis, -ism	condition
-itis	inflammation
-ize	to treat
-lith	stone
-lysis	disintegration, dissolution
-malacia	softening
-megaly	enlargement
-meter	measuring instrument
-oid	resemblance, likeness
-oma	tumor
-opathy, -pathy	any disease of
-orrhaphy	surgical repair
-osis	disease
-ostomy, -stomy	to form an opening
-otomy, -tomy	incision into
-penia	deficiency, decrease
-phage	ingesting
-phobia	fear

APPENDIX B

Sources of Scholarships and Loans

Johnson & Johnson has created a wonderful website to help promote careers in nursing. Go to www.discovernursing.com, and you will find lots of valuable information including hundreds of scholarships available to nursing students.

Don't forget to check with the financial aid office at your school. Then check out this list of state higher education agencies. They have information on education programs, colleges and universities, financial aid assistance programs, grants, scholarships, continuing education programs, and career opportunities.

Alabama Commission on Higher Education
PO Box 302000
Montgomery,
   AL 36130-2000
www.ache.state.al.us

Alaska Commission on Postsecondary Education
3030 Vintage Blvd
Juneau, AK 99801-7100
www.alaskadvantage.state.ak.us

Arizona Commission for Postsecondary Education
2020 North Central Ave,
   Suite 650
Phoenix, AZ 85004-4503
www.azhighered.gov/home.aspx

Arkansas Department of Higher Education
114 East Capitol
Little Rock,
   AR 72201-3818
www.adhe.arknet.edu

California Student Aid Commission
PO Box 419026
Rancho Cordova,
   CA 95741-9026
www.csac.ca.gov

Colorado Commission on Higher Education
1560 Broadway,
   Suite 1600
Denver, CO 80202
www.highered.colorado.gov

Connecticut Department of Higher Education
61 Woodland St
Hartford, CT 06105-1310
www.ctdhe.org

Delaware Higher Education Commission
Carvel State Office
   Building, 5th Floor
820 North French St
Wilmington, DE 19801
www.doe.k12.de.us/programs/dhec

District of Columbia
Office of the State
   Superintendent of
   Education State Board
   of Education
441 Fourth St NW,
   Suite 350 North
Washington, DC 20001
www.seo.dc.gov/seo/site/default.asp

Florida Office of Student Financial Assistance
State Department of
   Education
1940 North Monroe St,
   Suite 70
Tallahassee,
   FL 32303-4759
www.floridastudent-financialaid.org/osfahomepg.htm

Georgia Student Finance Commission State Loans and Grants Division
2082 East Exchange Pl
Tucker, GA 30084
www.gsfc.org

**Hawaii State
    Postsecondary
    Education Commission**
Office of the Board of
    Regents
2444 Dole St, Room 209
Honolulu, HI 96822-2302
www.hawaii.edu/offices/
    bor

Idaho Board of Education
PO Box 83720
650 West State St
Boise, ID 83720-0027
www.boardofed.idaho.gov

**Illinois Student
    Assistance
    Commission**
1755 Lake Cook Rd
Deerfield, IL 60015-5209
www.collegezone.com

**State Student Assistance
    Commission of Indiana**
150 West Market St,
    Suite 500
Indianapolis,
    IN 46204-2811
www.ssaci.in.gov

**Indiana Commission for
    Higher Education**
101 West Ohio St,
    Suite 550
Indianapolis,
    IN 46204-1984
www.che.in.gov

**Iowa College Student
    Aid Commission**
200 10th St, 4th Floor
Des Moines, IA 50309
www.iowacollegeaid.gov

Kansas Board of Regents
Curtis State Office Building
1000 SW Jackson St,
    Suite 520
Topeka, KS 66612-1368
www.kansasregents.org

**Kentucky Higher
    Education Assistance
    Authority**
PO Box 798
Frankfort, KY 40602-0798
www.kheaa.com

**Louisiana Office
    of Student Financial
    Assistance**
PO Box 91202
Baton Rouge,
    LA 70821-9202
www.osfa.la.gov

**Maine Education
    Assistance Division**
Finance Authority of Maine
PO Box 949
5 Community Dr
Augusta, ME 04332-0949
www.famemaine.com

**Maryland Higher
    Education Commission**
839 Bestgate Rd,
    Suite 400
Annapolis,
    MD 21401-3013
www.mhec.state.md.us

**Massachusetts
    Department of Higher
    Education**
One Ashburton Pl,
    Room 1401
Boston, MA 02108-1696
www.mass.edu

**Massachusetts Higher
    Education Information
    Center**
TERI College Planning
    Center
Boston Public Library
700 Boylston St
Boston, MA 02116
www.tericollegeplanning.org

**Michigan Student
    Financial Services
    Bureau**
Office of Scholarships and
    Grants
PO Box 30047
Lansing, MI 48909-7547
www.michigan.gov/
    mistudentaid

**Minnesota Office
    of Higher Education**
1450 Energy Park Dr,
    Suite 350
Saint Paul,
    MN 55108-5227
www.ohe.state.mn.us

**Mississippi Institutions
    of Higher Learning**
3825 Ridgewood Rd
Jackson, MS 39211-6453
www.ihl.state.ms.us

**Missouri Department
    of Higher Education**
3515 Amazonas Dr
Jefferson City,
    MO 65109-5717
www.dhe.mo.gov

**Montana University
    System**
2500 Broadway
PO Box 203201
Helena, MT 59620-3103
www.mus.edu

Nebraska Coordinating Commission for Postsecondary Education
140 North Eighth St, Suite 300
PO Box 95005
Lincoln, NE 68509-5005
www.ccpe.state.ne.us/ PublicDoc/CCPE/ Default.asp

Nevada Financial Aid Office
University of Nevada–Reno
Room 300 TSSC
Reno, NV 89557
www.finaid.unr.edu/ mainpage.htm

New Hampshire Postsecondary Education Commission
Three Barrell Court, Suite 300
Concord, NH 03301-8543
www.state.nh.us/ postsecondary

New Jersey Higher Education Student Assistance Authority
Quakerbridge Plaza, Building 4
Trenton, NJ 08625-0540
www.hesaa.org

New Jersey Commission on Higher Education
20 West State St
PO Box 542
www.state.nj.us/higheredu cation/index.htm

New Mexico Commission on Higher Education
1068 Cerrillos Rd
Santa Fe, NM 87505-1650
www.hed.state.nm.us

New York State Higher Education Services Corp.
99 Washington Ave
Albany, NY 12255
www.hesc.com

North Carolina State Education Assistance Authority
PO Box 13663
Research Triangle Park, NC 27709-3663
www.cfnc.org

North Dakota University System
North Dakota Student Financial Assistance Program
Department 215
600 East Boulevard Ave
Bismarck, ND 58505-0230
www.ndus.edu

Ohio Board of Regents
State Grants and Scholarships Department
PO Box 182452
Columbus, OH 43218-2452
www.regents.ohio.gov

Oklahoma State Regents for Higher Education
Oklahoma Guaranteed Student Loan Program
655 Research Pkwy, Suite 200
Oklahoma, OK 73104
www.okhighered.org

Oregon Student Assistance Commission
1500 Valley River Dr, Suite 100
Eugene, OR 97401
www.osac.state.or.us

Oregon University System
PO Box 3175
Eugene, OR 97403-0175
www.ous.edu

Pennsylvania Higher Education Assistance Agency
1200 North Seventh St
Harrisburg, PA 17102-1444
www.pdehighered.state. pa.us/higher/site/ default.asp

Office of Postsecondary and Higher Education (Pennsylvania)
State Department of Education
333 Market St, 12th Floor
Harrisburg, PA 17126-0333
www.pdehighered.state. pa.us/higher/site/ default.asp

Rhode Island Higher Education Assistance Authority
560 Jefferson Blvd, Suite 100
Warwick, RI 02886-1304
www.riheaa.org

Rhode Island Office of Higher Education
The Hazard Building
74 West Rd
Cranston, RI 02920
www.ribghe.org

South Carolina Commission on Higher Education
1333 Main St, Suite 200
Columbia, SC 29201
www.che.sc.gov

**South Dakota Board
of Regents**
306 East Capitol Ave,
Suite 200
Pierre, SD 57501
www.sdbor.edu

**Tennessee Higher
Education Commission**
Parkway Towers,
Suite 1900
404 James Robertson Pkwy
Nashville, TN 37243-6230
www.state.tn.us/thec

**Texas Higher Education
Coordinating Board**
PO Box 12788
Austin, TX 78711
www.thecb.state.tx.us

**Utah System of Higher
Education**
State Board of Regents
60 South 400 West
Salt Lake City,
UT 84101-1284
www.utahsbr.edu

**Vermont Student
Assistance Corporation**
10 East Allen St
PO Box 2000
Winooski, VT 05404-2601
services.vsac.org/ilwwcm/
connect/VSAC

**State Council of Higher
Education for Virginia**
James Monroe Building,
9th Floor
101 North 14th St
Richmond, VA 23219
www.schev.edu

**Washington State Higher
Education Coordinating
Board**
917 Lakeridge Way
PO Box 43430
Olympia, WA 98504-3430
www.hecb.wa.gov

**West Virginia Higher
Education Policy
Commission**
1018 Kanawha Blvd,
East Suite 700
Charleston, WV 25301
wvhepcnew.wvnet.edu

**Wisconsin Higher
Educational Aids Board**
131 West Wilson St,
Room 902
Madison, WI 53707-7885
www.heab.state.wi.us

**Wyoming Community
College Commission**
2020 Carey Ave, 8th Floor
Cheyenne, WY 82002
www.commission.wcc.edu

Territories

American Samoa
Board of Higher Education
(American Samoa)
American Samoa
Community College
PO Box 2609
Pago Pago, AS 96799
www.amsamoa.edu

**Commonwealth of the
Northern Mariana
Islands**
Northern Marianas College
Office of the President
PO Box 501250
Saipan, MP 96950-1250
www.nmcnet.edu

Puerto Rico
Council on Higher
Education (Puerto Rico)
PO Box 19900
San Juan, PR 00910-1900
www.ces.gobierno.pr

**Republic of the
Marshall Islands**
Scholarship Grant and
Loan Board (Republic
of the Marshall Islands)
PO Box 1436
Majuro, MH 96960
www.rmischolarship.net

Virgin Islands
Virgin Islands Department
of Education
Charlotte Amalie
1834 Kongens Gade
St. Thomas, VI 00801
www.doe.vi

APPENDIX C

State Nurses Associations

American Nurses Association
8515 Georgia Ave,
Suite 400
Silver Spring, MD 20910
www.nursingworld.org

Alabama State Nurses' Association
360 North Hull St.
Montgomery,
AL 36104-3658
www.alabamanurses.org

Alaska Nurses Association
3701 East Tudor Rd,
Suite 208
Anchorage,
AK 99507-1069
www.aknurse.org

Arizona Nurses Association
1850 E. Southern Ave,
Suite 1
Tempe, AZ 85282
www.aznurse.org

Arkansas Nurses Association
1123 S. University Ave,
#1015
Little Rock, AR 72204
www.arna.org

ANA–California
1121 L St, Suite 409
Sacramento, CA 95814
www.anacalifornia.org

Colorado Nurses Association
1221 South Clarkson St,
Suite 205
Denver, CO 80210
www.nurses-co.org

Connecticut Nurses Association
377 Research Pkwy,
Suite 2D
Meriden, CT 06450
www.ctnurses.org

Delaware Nurses Association
5586 Kirkwood Hwy
Wilmington, DE 19808
www.denurses.org

District of Columbia Nurses Association, Inc.
5100 Wisconsin Ave NW,
Suite 306
Washington, DC 20016
www.dcna.org

Federal Nurses Association
8515 Georgia Ave,
Suite 400
Silver Spring, MD 20910
www.fedna.org

Florida Nurses Association
PO Box 536985
Orlando, FL 32853-6985
www.floridanurse.org

Georgia Nurses Association
3032 Briarcliff Rd NE
Atlanta, GA 30329-2655
www.georgianurses.org

Guam Nurses Association
PO Box CG
Hagatna, Guam 96932
guamnurses@yahoo.com

Hawaii Nurses Association
677 Ala Moana Blvd,
Suite 301
Honolulu, HI 96813
www.hawaiinurses.org

Idaho Nurses Association
3525 Piedmont Rd NE
Building 5, Suite 300
Atlanta, GA 30305
www.idahonurses.org

Illinois Nurses Association
105 West Adams St,
Suite 2101
Chicago, IL 60603
www.illinoisnurses.com

Indiana State Nurses Association
2915 North High School Rd
Indianapolis, IN 46224
www.indiananurses.org

Iowa Nurses Association
1501 42nd St, Suite 471
West Des Moines,
IA 50266
www.iowanurses.org

Kansas State Nurses Association
1109 SW Topeka Blvd
Topeka, KS 66612
www.nursingworld.org/
snas/ks

Kentucky Nurses Association
PO Box 2616
Louisville, KY 40201-2616
www.kentucky-nurses.org

Louisiana State Nurses Association
5713 Superior Dr,
  Suite A-6
Baton Rouge, LA 70816
www.lsna.org

ANA–Maine
647 US Route 1, Suite 14
PMB #280
York, ME 03909
www.anamaine.org

Maryland Nurses Association
21 Governor's Ct,
  Suite 195
Baltimore, MD 21244
www.marylandrn.org

Massachusetts Association of Registered Nurses
PO Box 285
Milton, MA 02186
www.marnonline.org

Michigan Nurses Association
2310 Jolly Oak Rd
Okemos, MI 48864-4599
www.minurses.org

Minnesota Nurses Association
1625 Energy Park Dr,
  Suite 200
St. Paul, MN 55108
www.mnnurses.org

Mississippi Nurses Association
31 Woodgreen Pl
Madison, MS 39110
www.msnurses.org

Missouri Nurses Association
1904 Bubba Ln
Jefferson City,
  MO 65110-5228
www.missourinurses.org

Montana Nurses Association
20 Old Montana State Hwy
Clancy, MT 59634
www.mtnurses.org

Nebraska Nurses Association
PO Box 82086
Lincoln, NE 68508
www.nebraskanurses.org

Nevada Nurses Association
PO Box 34660
Reno, NV 89533
www.nvnurses.org

New Hampshire Nurses Association
210 N State St, Suite 1-A
Concord, NH 03301-3595
www.nhnurses.org

New Jersey State Nurses Association
1479 Pennington Rd
Trenton, NJ 08618-2661
www.njsna.org

New Mexico Nurses Association
PO Box 29658
Santa Fe,
  NM 87592-9658
www.nmna.org

New York State Nurses Association
11 Cornell Rd
Latham, NY 12110
www.nysna.org

North Carolina Nurses Association
103 Enterprise St,
  Box 12025
Raleigh, NC 27605
www.ncnurses.org

North Dakota Nurses Association
531 Airport Rd, Suite D
Bismarck,
  ND 58504-6107
www.ndna.org

Ohio Nurses Association
4000 East Main St
Columbus,
  OH 43213-2983
www.ohnurses.org

Oklahoma Nurses Association
6414 North Santa Fe,
  Suite A
Oklahoma City, OK 73116
www.oklahomanurses.org

Oregon Nurses Association
18765 SW Boones Ferry Rd
Tualatin, OR 97062
www.oregonrn.org

Pennsylvania State Nurses Association
2578 Interstate Dr,
  Suite 101
Harrisburg,
  PA 17110-9601
www.panurses.org

Rhode Island State Nurses Association
67 Park Place
Pawtucket, RI 02860
www.risnarn.org

South Carolina Nurses Association
1821 Gadsden St
Columbia, SC 29201
www.scnurses.org

South Dakota Nurses Association
116 N Euclid,
PO Box 1015
Pierre, SD 57501-1015
www.sdnursesassociation.org

Tennessee Nurses Association
545 Mainstream Dr,
Suite 405
Nashville, TN 37228-1201
www.tnaonline.org

Texas Nurses Association
7600 Burnet Rd,
Suite 440
Austin, TX 78757-1292
www.texasnurses.org

Utah Nurses Association
4505 South Wasatch Blvd,
#135
Salt Lake City, UT 84124
www.utahnursesassociation.com

Vermont State Nurses Association
100 Dorset St, Suite 13
South Burlington,
VT 05403-6241
www.vsna-inc.org

Virgin Islands State Nurses Association
PO Box 3617
Christiansted, US Virgin
Islands 00822

Virginia Nurses Association
7113 Three Chopt Rd,
Suite 204
Richmond, VA 23226
www.virginianurses.com

Washington State Nurses Association
575 Andover Park West,
Suite 101
Seattle, WA 98188-3321
www.wsna.org

West Virginia Nurses Association
PO 1946
405 Capitol St, Suite 600
Charleston, WV 25301
www.wvnurses.org

Wisconsin Nurses Association
6117 Monona Dr
Madison, WI 53716
www.wisconsinnurses.org

Wyoming Nurses Association
PMB Box 101
501 S Douglas Hwy,
Suite A
Gillette, WY 82716
www.wyonurse.org

APPENDIX D

Canadian Nurses Associations

Canadian Nurses Association
50 Driveway
Ottawa, Ontario K2P 1E2
www.cna-nurses.ca/cna

Canadian Nursing Students' Association
Fifth Avenue Court
99 Fifth Ave, Suite 15
Ottawa, Ontario K1S 5K4
www.cnsa.ca

Aboriginal Nurses Association of Canada
56 Sparks St, Suite 502
Ottawa, Ontario K1P 5A9
www.anac.on.ca

College & Association of Registered Nurses of Alberta
11620 168th St
Edmonton, Alberta
T5M 4A6
www.nurses.ab.ca

Association of Nurses of Prince Edward Island
53 Grafton St
Charlottetown, Prince
Edward Island C1A 1K8
www.arnpei.ca

Association of Registered Nurses of Newfoundland
55 Military Rd, Box 6116
St. Johns, Newfoundland
A1C 2C5
www.arnnl.nf.ca

Canadian Association for the History of Nursing
University of Alberta
114 89th Ave
Edmonton, Alberta
T6G 2M7
www.cahn-achn.ca

The Canadian Intravenous Nurses Association
PO Box 66572
685 McCowan Rd
Toronto, Ontario M1J 3N8
www.isips.org/cina.php

Canadian Nurses Foundation
50 Driveway
Ottawa, Ontario K2P 1E2
www.cnf-fiic.ca

College of Nurses of Ontario
101 Davenport Rd
Toronto, Ontario M5R 3P1
www.cno.org

College of Registered Nurses of Nova Scotia
7071 Bayers Rd,
Suite 4005
Halifax, NS B3L 2C2
www.cmns.ca

College of Registered Nurses of Manitoba
890 Pembina Hwy
Winnipeg, Manitoba
R3M 2M8
www.crnm.mb.ca

Registered Nurses Association of Northwest Territories and Nunavut
PO Box 2757
Yellowknife, Northwest
Territories X1A 2R1
www.rnantnu.ca

Nurse Association of New Brunswick
165 Regent St
Fredericton, New
Brunswick E3B 7B4
www.nanb.nb.ca

Ontario Nurses' Association
85 Grenville St, Suite 400
Toronto, Ontario M5S 3A2
www.ona.org

Order of Nurses of the Province of Quebec
4200 Dorchester Blvd W
Montreal, Quebec
H3Z 1V4
www.oiiq.org

College of Registerted Nurses of British Columbia
2855 Arbutus St
Vancouver, British
Columbia V6J 3Y8
www.crnbc.ca

Registered Nurses Association of Ontario
158 Pearl St
Toronto, Ontario M5H 1L3
www.rnao.org

Saskatchewan Registered Nurses' Association
2066 Retallack St
Regina, Saskatchewan
S4T 7X5
www.srna.org

United Nurses of Alberta
10611 98th Ave, #900
Edmonton, Alberta
T5K 2P7
www.una.ab.ca

Yukon Nurses Society
204-4133 4th Ave
Whitehorse, Yukon
Y1A 1H8
www.yrna.ca

Specialty Nursing Organizations

**Academy of Medical-
Surgical Nurses**
E Holly Ave, Box 56
Pitman, NJ 08071-0056
www.medsurgnurse.org

**Air & Surface Transport
Nurses Association**
7995 East Prentice Ave,
Suite 100
Greenwood Village,
CO 80111
www.astna.org

**American Academy
of Ambulatory Care
Nursing**
E Holly Ave, Box 56
Pitman, NJ 08071-0056
www.aaacn.org

**American Academy
of Nurse Practitioners**
PO Box 12846
Austin, TX 78711
www.aanp.org

**American Academy
of Nursing**
888 17th St, NW
Suite 800
Washington, DC 20006
www.aannet.org

**American Academy
of Wound Management**
1155 15th St NW,
Suite 500
Washington, DC 20005
www.aawm.org

**American Assembly
for Men in Nursing**
PO Box 130220
Birmingham, AL 35213
www.aamn.org

**American Association for
the History of Nursing**
10200 W 44th Ave,
Suite 304
Wheat Ridge, CO 80033
www.aahn.org

**American Association
of Colleges of Nursing**
1 Dupont Circle, NW,
Suite 530
Washington, DC 20036
www.aacn.nche.edu

**American Association
of Critical-Care Nurses**
101 Columbia
Aliso Viejo,
CA 92656-4109
www.aacn.org

**American Association
of Diabetes Educators**
200 W Madison St,
Suite 800
Chicago, IL 60606
www.aadenet.org

**American Association
of Legal Nurse
Consultants**
401 N Michigan Ave
Chicago, IL 60611
www.aalnc.org

**The American Association
of Managed Care
Nurses, Inc.**
4435 Waterfront Dr,
Suite 101
Glen Allen, VA 23060
www.aamcn.org

**American Association
of Neuroscience
Nurses**
4700 W Lake Ave
Glenview, IL 60025
www.aann.org

**American Association
of Nurse Anesthetists**
222 S Prospect Ave
Park Ridge,
IL 60068-4001
www.aana.com

**The American Association
of Nurse Attorneys**
TAANA
PO Box 515
Coumbus,
OH 43216-0515
www.taana.org

**American Association
of Occupational Health
Nurses, Inc.**
2920 Brandywine Rd,
Suite 100
Atlanta, GA 30341
www.aaohn.org

**American Association
of Office Nurses**
109 Kinderkamack Rd
Montvale, NJ 07645

**American Association
of Spinal Cord Injury
Nurses**
801 18th St NW
Washington, DC 20006
www.aascin.org

**American Board
of Nursing Specialties**
610 Thornhill Lane
Aurora, OH 44202
www.nursingcertification.
org

**American College
of Nurse Midwives**
8403 Colesville Rd,
Suite 1550
Silver Spring, MD 20910
www.midwife.org

**American College
of Nurse Practitioners**
1501 Wilson Blvd,
Suite 509
Arlington, VA 22209
www.acnpweb.org

American Forensic Nurses
225 N El Cielo Rd,
Suite 195
Palm Springs, CA 92262
www.amrn.com

**American Holistic Nurses
Association**
323 N San Francisco St,
Suite 201
Flagstaff, AZ 86001
www.ahna.org

**American Long Term Care
Nurses Association**
11427 Reed Hartman Hwy
Cincinnati, OH 45241
www.alsna.com

**American Nephrology
Nurses' Association**
E Holly Ave, Box 56
Pitman, NJ 08071-0056
www.annanurse.org

**American Organization
of Nurse Executives**
1 N Franklin, 32nd floor
Chicago, IL 60606
www.aone.org

**American Psychiatric
Nurses Association**
1555 Wilson Blvd,
Suite 530
Arlington, VA 22209
www.apna.org

**American Radiological
Nurses Association**
820 Jorie Blvd
Oak Brook, IL 60523-2251
www.rsna.org

**American Association for
Long-Term Care Nurses**
11427 Reed Hartman Hwy
Cincinnati, OH 45421
www.ltcnursing.org

**American Society for Pain
Management Nursing**
PO Box 15473
Lenexa, KS 66285-5473
www.aspmn.org

**American Society of
PeriAnesthesia Nurses**
10 Melrose Ave, Suite 110
Cherry Hill, NJ 08003-3696
www.aspan.org

**American Society
of Plastic and
Reconstructive
Surgical Nurses**
7794 Grow Dr
Pensacola, FL 32514
www.aspsn.org

**Association for
Professionals in
Infection Control and
Epidemiology, Inc.**
1275 K St NW, Suite 1000
Washington,
DC 20005-4006
www.apic.org

**Association of Nurses
in AIDS Care**
3538 Ridgewood Rd
Akron, OH 44333-3122
www.anacnet.org

**Association of Pediatric
Oncology Nurses**
4700 W Lake Ave
Glenview, IL 60025-1485
www.apon.org

**Association of
Perioperative
Registered Nurses**
2170 S Parker Rd,
Suite 300
Denver, CO 80231-5711
www.aorn.org

**Association of
Rehabilitation Nurses**
4700 W Lake Ave
Glenview, IL 60025-1485
www.rehabnurse.org

Association of Women's Health, Obstetric and Neonatal Nurses
2000 L St NW, Suite 740
Washington, DC 20036
www.awhonn.org

Case Management Society of America
6301 Ranch Dr
Little Rock, AR 72223
www.cmsa.org

Chi Eta Phi Sorority, Inc.
3029 Thirteenth St NW
Washington, DC 20009
www.chietaphi.com

Emergency Nurses Association
915 Lee St
Des Plaines,
IL 60016-6569
www.ena.org

Endocrine Nurses Society
PO Box 21106
Milwaukee WI. 5322
www.endo-nurses.org

National Association for Home Care & Hospice
228 Seventh St SE
Washington, DC 20003
www.nahc.org

Hospice and Palliative Nurses Association
Penn Center West One,
Suite 229
Pittsburgh, PA 15276
www.hpna.org

Infusion Nurses Society
315 Norwood Park S
Norwood, MA 02062
www.ins1.org

International Council of Nurses
3, Place Jean Marteau
1201-Geneva
Switzerland
www.icn.ch

International Society of Nurses in Genetics
461 Cochran Rd, Box 246
Pittsburgh, PA 15228
www.isong.org

International Transplant Nurses Society
1739 E Carson St, Box 351
Pittsburgh, PA 15203-1700
www.itns.org

League of Intravenous Therapy Education
Empire Bldg, Suite 3
3001 Jacks Run Rd
White Oak, PA 15131
www.lite.org

National Alliance of Nurse Practitioners
325 Pennsylvania Ave SE,
PMB 350
Washington,
DC 20003-1100
www.medpedia.com/groups/66-NP

National Association of Clinical Nurse Specialists
2090 Linglestown Rd,
Suite 107
Harrisburg, PA 17110
www.nacns.org

National Association of Hispanic Nurses
1455 Pennsylvania Ave,
NW, Suite 400
Washington, DC 20004
www.thehispanicnurses.org

National Association of Neonatal Nurses
4700 W Lake Ave
Glenview, IL 60025-1485
www.nann.org

National Association of Nurse Massage Therapists
28 Lowry Dr
PO Box 232
West Milton, OH 45383
www.nanmt.org

National Association of Orthopaedic Nurses
401 N Michigan Ave,
Suite 2200
Chicago, IL 60611
www.orthonurse.org

National Association of Pediatric Nurse Associates & Practitioners, Inc.
20 Brace Rd, Suite 200
Cherry Hill,
NJ 08034-2634
www.napnap.org

National Association of School Nurses
8484 Georgia Ave,
Suite 420
Silver Spring, MD 20910
www.nasn.org

National Association of Subacute/Post Acute Care
624 Dresden Ave
East Liverpool,
Ohio 43920
www.naspac.net

Association for Vascular Access
5526 West 13400 South, Suite 229
Herriman, UT 84096
www.avainfo.org

National Black Nurses Association, Inc.
8630 Fenton St, Suite 330
Silver Spring,
MD 20910-3803
www.nbna.org

National Coalition of Ethnic Minority Nurse Associations
6101 West Centinela Ave, Suite 378
Culver City, CA 90230
www.ncemna.org

National Council of State Boards of Nursing, Inc.
111 East Wacker Dr, Suite 2900
Chicago, IL 60601
www.ncsbn.org

National Federation of Licensed Practical Nurses, Inc.
605 Poole Dr
Garner, NC 27529
www.nflpn.org

National Gerontological Nursing Association
7794 Grow Dr
Pensacola, FL 32514
www.ngna.org

National League for Nursing
61 Broadway, 33rd Floor
New York, NY 10006
www.nln.org

International Nurses Society on Addictions
PO Box 163635
Columbus, OH 43216
www.intnsa.org

National Nursing Staff Development Organization
7794 Grow Dr
Pensacola, FL 32514
www.nnsdo.org

National Organization for Associate Degree Nursing
7794 Grow Dr
Pensacola, FL 32514
www.noadn.org

National Student Nurses' Association
45 Main St, Suite 606
Brooklyn, NY 11201
www.nsna.org

Nurses Christian Fellowship
Box 7895
Madison, WI 53707-7895
www.ncf-jcn.org

Oncology Nursing Society
125 Enterprise Dr
Pittsburgh, PA 15275
www.ons.org

Philippine Nurses Association of America, Inc
20127 Avenida Pamplona
Cerritos, CA 90703
www.philippinenursesaa.org

Respiratory Nursing Society
309 E Lee Ave
Vinton, VA 24179
www.respiratorynursing-society.org

Sigma Theta Tau International Honor Society of Nursing
550 W North St
Indianapolis, IN 46202
www.nursingsociety.org

Society for Vascular Nursing
203 Washington St, PMB 311
Salem, MA 01970
www.svnnet.org

Society of Gastroenterology Nurses and Associates, Inc.
401 North Michigan Ave
Chicago, IL 60611-4267
www.sgna.org

Society of Otorhinolaryngology and Head-Neck Nurses, Inc.
202 Julia St
New Smyrna Beach, FL 32168
www.sohnnurse.com

Society of Urologic Nurses and Associates
E Holly Ave, Box 56
Pitman, NJ 08071-0056
www.suna.org

**Transcultural Nursing
  Society**
Madonna University
36600 Schoolcraft Rd
Livonia, MI 48150-1173
www.tcns.org

**Visiting Nurse
  Associations
  of America**
900 19th St,
  NW Suite 200
Washington, DC 20006
www.vnaa.org

**Wound, Ostomy and
  Continence Nurses
  Society**
15000 Commerce Pkwy,
  Suite C
Mt. Laurel, NJ 08054
www.wocn.org

APPENDIX F

U.S. State and Territorial Boards of Nursing

Alabama Board of Nursing
770 Washington Ave
RSA Plaza, Suite 250
Montgomery,
 AL 36130-3900
www.abn.state.al.us

Alaska Board of Nursing
Robert B. Atwood Building
550 W 7th Ave,
 Suite 1500
Anchorage, AK 99501
www.dced.state.ak.us/occ/
 pnur.htm

**American Samoa
 Health Services**
Regulatory Board
LBJ Tropical Medical Center
Pago Pago, AS 96799

**Arizona State Board
 of Nursing**
4747 North 7th St,
 Suite 200
Phoenix, AZ 85014
www.azbn.gov

**Arkansas State Board
 of Nursing**
University Tower Building
1123 S University,
 Suite 800
Little Rock,
 AR 72204-1619
www.state.ar.us/nurse

**California Board
 of Registered Nursing**
Board of Registered Nursing
PO Box 944210
Sacramento,
 CA 94244-2100
www.rn.ca.gov

Colorado Board of Nursing
1560 Broadway,
 Suite 1350
Denver, CO 80202
www.dora.state.co.us/
 nursing

**Connecticut Board
 of Nursing**
410 Capitol Ave,
 PO Box 340308
Hartford, CT 06134-0308
www.state.ct.us/dph

**Delaware Board
 of Nursing**
861 Silver Lake Blvd
Cannon Building,
 Suite 203
Dover, DE 19904
dpr.delaware.gov/boards/
 nursing/index.shtml

**District of Columbia
 Board of Nursing**
Department of Health
825 N Capitol St NE,
 2nd Floor, Room 2224
Washington, DC 20002
www.dchealth.dc.gov

Florida Board of Nursing
4052 Bald Cypress Way,
 BIN C02
Tallahasseee,
 FL 32399-3252
www.doh.state.fl.us/mqa/
 nursing/nur_home.html

Georgia Board of Nursing
237 Coliseum Dr
Macon, GA 31217-3858
www.sos.georgia.gov/PLB/
 RN

**Guam Board of Nurse
 Examiners**
PO Box 2816
Agana, Guam 96932

Hawaii Board of Nursing
Professional & Vocational
 Licensing Division
PO Box 3469
Honolulu, HI 96801
www.hawaii.gov/dcca/areas/
 pvl/boards/nursing

Idaho Board of Nursing
280 N 8th St, Suite 210
Boise, ID 83720
www2.state.id.us/ibn

**Illinois Department
 of Professional
 Regulation**
320 W Washington
Springfield, IL 62786
www/state.il.us/dpr

**Indiana State Board
 of Nursing**
Health Professions Bureau
402 W Washington St,
 Room W041
Indianapolis, IN 46204
www.state.in.us/
 hpb/boards/isbn

Iowa Board of Nursing
River Point Business Park
400 SW 8th St, Suite B
Des Moines,
 IA 50309-4685
www.state.ia.us/
 government/nursing/
 index.htm

**Kansas State Board
of Nursing**
Landon State Office
  Building
900 SW Jackson,
  Suite 551-S
Topeka, KS 66612-1230
www.ksbn.org

**Kentucky Board
of Nursing**
312 Whittington Pkwy,
  Suite 300
Louisville, KY 40222
www.kbn.ky.gov

**Louisiana State Board
of Nursing**
3510 N Causeway Blvd,
  Suite 501
Metairie, LA 70003
www.lsbn.state.la.us

**Maine State Board
of Nursing**
158 State House Station
Augusta, ME 04333
www.maine.gov/
  boardofnursing

**Maryland Board
of Nursing**
4140 Patterson Ave
Baltimore, MD 21215
www.mbon.org

**Massachusetts Board
of Registration
in Nursing**
Commonwealth of
  Massachusetts
239 Causeway St
Boston, MA 02114
www.state.ma.us/
  reg/boards/rn

**Michigan CIS/Office
of Health Services**
Ottawa Towers North
611 W Ottawa, 4th Floor
Lansing, MI 48933
www.michigan.gov/
  healthlicense

**Minnesota Board
of Nursing**
2829 University Ave SE,
  Suite 200
Minneapolis, MN 55414
www.nursingboard.state.
  mn.us

**Mississippi Board
of Nursing**
1935 Lakeland Dr, Suite B
Jackson, MS 39216-5014
www.msbn.state.ms.us

**Missouri State Board
of Nursing**
3605 Missouri Blvd
Jefferson City,
  MO 65102-0656
www.pr.mo.gov

Montana Board of Nursing
301 South Park
Helena, MT 59620-0513
mt.gov/dli/nur

**Nebraska Health
and Human Services
System**
Dept of Regulation
  & Licensure, Nursing
  Section
301 Centennial Mall S
Lincoln, NE 68509-4986
www.hhs.state.ne.us

**Nevada State Board
of Nursing**
License Certification
  and Education
4330 S Valley View Blvd,
  Suite 106
Las Vegas, NV 89103
www.nursingboard.
  state.nv.us

**New Hampshire Board
of Nursing**
79 Regional Dr, Bldg B
Concord, NH 03301
www.nh.gov/nursing

**New Jersey Board
of Nursing**
PO Box 45010
124 Halsey St, 6th Floor
Newark, NJ 07101
www.state.nj.us/lps/ca/
  medical.htm

**New Mexico Board
of Nursing**
4206 Louisiana Blvd NE,
  Suite A
Albuquerque, NM 87109
www.bon.state.nm.us

**New York State Board
of Nursing**
Education Bldg
89 Washington Ave
2nd Floor West Wing
Albany, NY 12234
www.op.nysed.gov/
  nurse.htm

**North Carolina Board
of Nursing**
3724 National Dr,
  Suite 201
Raleigh, NC 27612
www.ncbon.com

**North Dakota Board
of Nursing**
919 S 7th St, Suite 504
Bismarck, ND 58504
www.ndbon.org

Northern Mariana Islands
Commonwealth Board
of Nurse Examiners
PO Box 501458
Saipan, MP 96950

Ohio Board of Nursing
17 South High St,
Suite 400
Columbus,
OH 43215-3413
www.nursing.ohio.gov

**Oklahoma Board
of Nursing**
2915 N Classen Blvd,
Suite 524
Oklahoma City, OK 73106
www.ok.gov/nursing

**Oregon State Board
of Nursing**
800 NE Oregon St, Box 25
Suite 465
Portland, OR 97232
www.osbn.state.or.us

**Pennsylvania State Board
of Nursing**
PO Box 2649
124 Pine St
Harrisburg, PA 17105
www.dos.state.pa.us/
bpoa/nurbd/
mainpage.htm

**Puerto Rico Board
of Nurse Examiners**
800 Roberto H. Todd Ave,
Room 202, Stop 18
Santurce, PR 00908

**Rhode Island Board
of Nurse Registration
and Nursing Education**
105 Cannon Building
Three Capitol Hill
Providence, RI 02908
www.health.state.ri.us

**South Carolina State
Board of Nursing**
Synergy Business Park
Kingstree Building
110 Centerview Dr,
Suite 202
Columbia, SC 29210
www.lir.state.sc.us/pol/
nursing

**South Dakota Board
of Nursing**
4300 South Louise Ave,
Suite C-1
Sioux Falls,
SD 57106-3124
www.doh.sd.gov/boards/
nursing

**Tennessee State Board
of Nursing**
426 Fifth Ave North
1st Floor, Cordell
Hull Building
Nashville, TN 37247
www.health.state.tn.us/Bo
ards/nursing

**Texas Board of Nurse
Examiners**
333 Guadalupe,
Suite 3-460
Austin, TX 78701
www.bne.state.tx.us

**Utah Division
of Occupational
and Professional
Licensing**
Heber M. Wells Bldg,
4th Floor
160 East 300 South
Salt Lake City, UT 84111
www.dopl.utah.gov/
licensing/
nursing.html

**Vermont State Board
of Nursing**
109 State St
Montpelier,
VT 05609-1101
www.vtprofessionals.org/
opr1/nurses

**Virgin Islands Board
of Nurse Licensure**
Veterans Drive Station
St. Thomas, VI 00803
www.vibnl.org

Virginia Board of Nursing
6603 W Broad St,
5th Floor
Richmond, VA 23230
www.dhp.state.va.
us/Nursing

**Washington State Nursing
Care Quality Assurance
Commission**
Department of Health
Health Systems Quality
Assurance
310 Israel Rd
Tumwater, WA 98501
www.doh.wa.gov/hsqa/
professions/Nursing/
default.htm

**West Virginia Board
 of Examiners
 for Registered
 Professional Nurses**
101 Dee Dr
Charleston, WV 25311
www.wvrnboard.com

**West Virginia State
 Board of Examiners
 for Licensed Practical
 Nurses**
101 Dee Dr
Charleston,
   WV 25311-1620
www.lpnboard.state.wv.us

**Wisconsin Department
 of Regulation
 and Licensing**
1400 E Washington Ave
Madison, WI 53708
www.drl.wi.gov

**Wyoming State Board
 of Nursing**
2020 Carey Ave,
   Suite 110
Cheyenne, WY 82002
www.nursing.state.wy.us

APPENDIX G

Resources for NCLEX® Review Available from Mosby/Elsevier

For more information on these products and others, please visit our website at www.elsevier.com.

Illustrated Study Guide for the NCLEX-PN Exam, 7th edition
JoAnn Zerwekh and Jo Carol Claborn

With its concise outline format summarizing essential nursing content and multiple illustrations, including many of the authors' popular mnemonic cartoons, *Illustrated Study Guide for the NCLEX-PN Exam,* 7th edition is the perfect study companion for the NCLEX-PN exam. The colorful and user-friendly design includes a special Alert! feature highlighting frequently tested nursing concepts, and Nursing Priority boxes identifying priorities of care. The book also includes a review of the latest NCLEX test plan and new alternate item format questions, plus chapters on pharmacology, life span, basic nursing concepts, and body systems to provide the most complete study guide available for the NCLEX-PN exam. **ISBN: 978-0-323-03957-4**

Illustrated Study Guide for the NCLEX-RN Exam, 7th edition
JoAnn Zerwekh and Jo Carol Claborn

Fun and engaging, this must-have review resource covers the nursing concepts and content found on the latest NCLEX-RN examination. It features a concise outline format that's perfect for studying, as well as 2020 review questions to test your knowledge and help you prepare for the exam. Colorful illustrations and mnemonic cartoons clarify essential nursing concepts and offer a visual way for you to remember key facts for the NCLEX exam. Answers and rationales are provided for every practice question. **ISBN: 978-0-323-05664-9**

Mosby's Comprehensive Review of Practical Nursing for the NCLEX-PN Examination, 15th edition
Mary Eyles

Concise review outlines reinforce your knowledge of nursing fundamentals, pharmacology, and nutrition, and chapters on emergency, medical-surgical, pediatric, maternity/women's health, and mental health help you understand concepts as they relate to the exam. This essential guide also includes a multitude of review questions in a variety of NCLEX-style formats, plus two comprehensive sample exams that prepare you for the test-taking experience and ensure successful results! **ISBN: 978-0-323-04707-4**

Mosby's Comprehensive Review of Nursing for the NCLEX-RN Examination, 19th edition

Dolores F. Saxton, Patricia M. Nugent, and Phyllis K. Pelikan

This title is now completely reorganized and in full color for an even better studying experience! Content is divided into units covering the core areas of medical-surgical, pediatric, maternity/women's health, and mental health nursing. Smaller chapters within the units break down information into smaller, more manageable pieces for a complete review of key content. NCLEX-RN examination-style questions, including the newest alternate item formats, follow each unit and help you master the content and practice with critical thinking questions seen on the exam. With more than 4100 questions with rationales in the book and on the companion CD for practice in print and electronic formats, this all-inclusive review is a vital study tool for the NCLEX-RN exam. **ISBN: 978-0-323-05304-4**

Mosby's Review Cards for the NCLEX-RN Examination, 3rd edition

Martin S. Manno

This set of 450 review cards provides an easy way for students to study for the NCLEX-RN examination. It contains 1221 NCLEX exam-style questions, including the new alternate item formats. Organized by clinical area and body system, practice questions appear on the front of each card. The reverse side features each question's answer, rationale, cognitive level, nursing process step, and NCLEX test plan category. An overview of the latest NCLEX-RN test plan, preparation, and a comprehensive exam is also included in separate sections. **ISBN: 978-0-323-05742-4**

Mosby's Review Questions for the NCLEX-RN Examination, 6th edition

Dolores F. Saxton, Patricia M. Nugent, Phyllis K. Pelikan, and Judith S. Green

Mosby's Review Questions for the NCLEX-RN Examination, 6th edition is the practice tool you need to confidently prepare for the NCLEX-RN exam. This edition includes more than 5000 exam-style review questions designed to help you assess your strengths and weaknesses, enhance your clinical application skills, and reduce test anxiety. A companion CD included with every text familiarizes you with the electronic testing experience and provides instant feedback for enhanced study. **ISBN: 978-0-323-04724-1**

Mosby's PDQ for NCLEX-RN

Pocket-sized and easy to use, this study guide to the NCLEX-RN examination offers valuable test-taking strategies and tools. It's the only portable guide with a Question Dissector that breaks down sample questions to help you find the correct answer, by highlighting key terms and offering helpful hints along with answers and rationales. NCLEX exam-style questions include all types of alternate item formats such as multiple choice, Select All That Apply, Hot Spots, and Fill in the Blank questions. A mini CD gives students the opportunity to answer even more practice questions on the computer! **ISBN: 978-0-323-05419-5**

Mosby's RNtertainment: An NCLEX Review Board Game
Karen Trafton

Mosby's RNtertainment: An NCLEX Review Board Game is a revolutionary game designed as a review tool for nursing students preparing for the NCLEX exam or for practicing nurses who want to reinforce and sharpen their nursing knowledge. It presents clinical questions and scenarios in all the major nursing categories while providing a fun, humorous, and innovative way to study. Perfect for study groups and gift giving, this game includes a colorful game board, unique die, game pieces, and color-coded category cards that are divided into the four main areas of Medication, Disease Process/Anatomy & Physiology, Diagnostic Testing, and Patient Care. Two wild card categories titled Healthy Rewards and Code Black and Blue also incorporate humorous patient scenarios into the game to test the will and ability of a nurse to "handle it all." The object of the game is to travel from start to finish by correctly answering nursing-related questions while navigating through the situations randomly faced in the Healthy Rewards and Code Black and Blue cards. **ISBN: 978-0-323-04480-6**

Saunders Comprehensive Review for the NCLEX-PN Examination, 4th edition
Linda Anne Silvestri

This truly unique, bestselling review and preparation resource offers the perfect combination of core content review, practice questions with comprehensive rationales, and detailed test-taking strategies and tips. Throughout the book you'll find Linda Silvestri's hallmark Pyramid to Success learning features that highlight key information, and more than 1000 high-quality review questions that mirror the latest NCLEX-PN test plan. The companion CD contains all of the questions from the book, plus more than 2600 additional practice questions in a flexible electronic format that allows you to customize your study experience and focus on those areas you need to review the most. **ISBN: 978-1-4160-4730-8**

Saunders Comprehensive Review for the NCLEX-RN Examination, 4th edition
Linda Anne Silvestri

This book and its accompanying CD provide students with more than 4200 practice questions. All questions include comprehensive rationales and test-taking strategies. The book covers all the nursing content tested on the NCLEX-RN exam and offers chapters on preparation for the NCLEX-RN exam from a student's perspective. The CD contains all 1800 multiple-choice questions from the book, plus more than 2200 additional practice questions not found in the text. **ISBN: 978-1-4160-3708-8**

Saunders Online Review Course for the NCLEX-RN Examination (offered in 4-, 8-, and 16-week versions)
Linda Anne Silvestri

Saunders Online Review Course for the NCLEX-RN Examination offers a comprehensive review of core nursing areas and more than 2000 review questions that will assess strengths and weaknesses, focus study time, and increase confidence. A diagnostic pretest identifies strengths and weaknesses and maps the individual student's course of study. Interactive lessons including animations, video clips, case studies, and mini quizzes and assessments highlight key concepts and reinforce learning.

Saunders Q&A Review Cards for the NCLEX-RN
Linda Anne Silvestri

The perfect companion to Saunders Comprehensive Review for the NCLEX-RN Examination, the Q&A Review Cards contain 1000 additional practice questions. Each question includes Silvestri's hallmark detailed rationales for both the correct and incorrect options, plus comprehensive test-taking strategies. The practice questions, which are organized according to the Client Needs identified on the 2007 Test Plan, appear on the front of each card. The reverse side features each question's answer, rationale, test-taking strategy, and integrated process. **ISBN: 978-1-4160-4726-1**

Saunders Q&A Review for the NCLEX-PN Examination, 4th edition
Linda Anne Silvestri

This text is written and organized to address specific Client Needs and Integrated Processes in the 2008 NCLEX-PN test plan. The text and accompanying CD contain 3200 practice questions—including all types of Alternate Item Format questions—that include comprehensive rationales for both correct and incorrect options, test-taking strategies for each question, and a textbook page reference for further explanation. The companion CD also provides computerized testing practice in study, quiz, or exam modes, and allows you to choose from 21 different content categories to focus your study sessions. **ISBN: 978-1-4160-6201-1**

Saunders Q&A Review for the NCLEX-RN Examination, 4th edition
Linda Anne Silvestri

More than 5200 NCLEX-RN examination-style questions each with rationales, test-taking strategies, and textbook page references for each question provide immediate feedback and make it easy to learn and understand the material. Plus you can study on the computer in three different modes—study, quiz, or exam—with the companion CD. **ISBN: 978-1-4160-4850-3**

Saunders Strategies for Success for the NCLEX-RN Examination

Linda Anne Silvestri

This text is a critical component of the Saunders Pyramid to Success review products for the NCLEX-RN examination. Whether this is the first or last review product purchased, this book will help students feel well prepared and confident as they prepare for the boards or any exam throughout the nursing curriculum. This book includes test-taking strategies for specific question types including true-false response, prioritization, communication, pharmacology, leadership, and delegation questions. A two-color design, open layout, and casual writing style make this book especially appealing to students. This book would be a great companion to any of the review and testing products currently on the market. **ISBN: 978-1-4160-0095-2**

Index

Note: Page number followed by *f* denotes figures, *t* denotes tables and *b* denotes boxes.